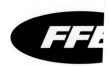 

GW00374025

Fit For Business
The Ultimate Competitive Edge

Rob Rowland-Smith
& Harry Hodge

The Blue Group

Edited and produced by Phil Jarratt
Designed by Paul Sheavils
Principal photography by Richard Bailey
Additional photography by Michael Simmons, Rennie Ellis, Afiff,
Phil Jarratt

A note from the publisher
All reasonable care and attention has been taken in the preparation of this book and the attached charts. It is not intended that the information herein should be used by the reader as a substitute for appropriate professional attention and medical care. The reader should first consult his or her doctor before beginning any program described herein, and the publisher, authors, consultants and editor, their respective employees and agents, shall not accept responsibility for any injury, loss or damage caused to any person acting or failing to act arising from the material in this book.

First published in Australia in 1999 by The Blue Group
ACN No 011 027 535
PO Box 321 Noosa Heads Q 4567 Australia
Phone: 61 7 5449 9087 Fax: 61 7 5449 0188
Email: bluegroup@peg.apc.org
http:/www.noosanetcafe.com.au/blue/

National Library of Australia Cataloguing-in-Publication data:
Fit For Business
The Ultimate Competitive Edge
Rowland-Smith, Rob and Hodge, Harry
ISBN 0-9587420-2-2

Printed in Hong Kong by Paramount Printing
Distributed in Australia by Tower Books (61 2 9975 5566)
Distributed in the UK by Turnaround (44 181 829 3000)

How to use this book

This book is your personal trainer. Within its pages you will find the complete guide to the Fit For Business five hour plan for health and fitness at the peak of your career.

Some assumptions have been made. The first is that you really want to improve your health and fitness. If only you had the time. This book will show you that you can make the time.

The second is that you recognise the correlation between physical and psychological fitness and understand the importance of the competitive edge in all walks of life. We make no apologies for the fact that Fit For Business is designed for achievers. Everyone can benefit from FFB, but those who will benefit most are those who understand the difference between adequacy and excellence.

We suggest you take the time to read the book through before turning to the seven wall charts which show you how to do the programs. The early chapters explain the physiology and the philosophy of FFB and its application to your life in work and play. The most important element in all these chapters is defined by one word - balance. FFB does not lay down laws no busy person can obey. Rather, it explains how health and fitness is an asset and your life is a balance sheet. FFB is simply business, and if you understand business, FFB will work for you.

In the second half of the book Rob Rowland-Smith explains the how and why of every exercise in each of the FFB programs, so that you can understand and monitor your own progress.

Finally, the seven charts within the book may be pulled out for the wall of your home gym or simply folded out so that you can follow the programs wherever you are. They represent your step-by-step guide to FFB's five hour plan to health and fitness.

FFB

Acknowledgements

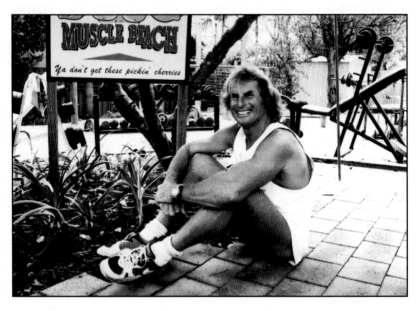

I would like to acknowledge the following:

1. Phil Jarratt for his expertise, his sense of humour and for adopting the FFB program himself. (Good on ya, Cyril.)

2. Harry Hodge for his dedication and commitment, but above all, for showing there is so much potential in all of us.

3. Paul Sheavils and the staff at The Blue Group for making this book a reality.

4. Richard Bailey for his excellent principal photography, and Michael Simmons, Rennie Ellis and Afiff for their photographic contributions.

5. The staff at the Sydney Academy of Sport's Human Performance Laboratory, Narrabeen, NSW, for co-ordinating and monitoring the fitness testing.

I'd like to dedicate this book to those I have taught, coached and trained over the years, to my friends and family, especially my wife Judy and my children, Rhiannon, Stefanie and Ryan.

And finally, to my other family, my family of sandhill warriors all over the world - you are the inspiration for what I do, and the reason I love doing it.

Rob Rowland-Smith

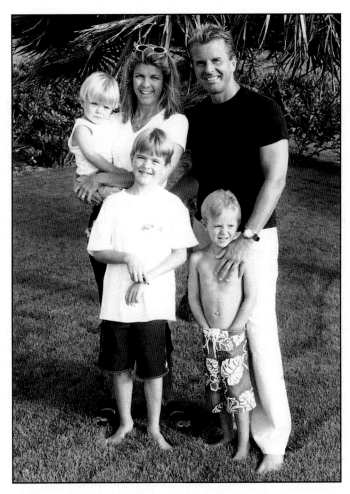

I would like to dedicate this book to all those people who aspire to a fit and healthy lifestyle.

I would also like to acknowledge and thank my family and friends for their support and encouragement in everything I do. Especially my wife, Sandee, for her contributions to this book as a participant in all the programs and the chart photos. I want to make mention of our three boys, Mathieu, Tommy and Ben, who give us inspiration and so much pleasure.

Lastly I want to thank my mother, Marcia Hodge, who provided the foundation in my life that every child needs - love, support and encouragement.

Harry Hodge

About the Authors

In a career in journalism, business and film which has seen dramatic highs and lows over the past 25 years, Quiksilver Europe CEO Harry Hodge has come to realise that when he is physically fit, he is fit for business.

"At three different stages of my life I've been out of shape and generally unhealthy, "says Hodge, now 49. "On each of these occasions I've been struggling with my business and my career. With the benefit of hindsight, I'm convinced that this was no coincidence. Health, fitness and success walk hand in hand."

This is the philosophy behind Fit For Business, a comprehensive fitness manual for busy people at the peak of their careers, co-authored by Hodge and fitness trainer Rob Rowland-Smith. Says Hodge: "In most people's careers, these are the peak performance years, the time of your life when you are busiest and when every decision is an important one. Unfortunately, too many executives let career pressure affect their levels of fitness. This book explains that no executive can afford to do that, because fitness is one of the keys to business success."

Fit, tanned, relaxed and in charge of a $US150 million France-based company whose growth curve in the 1990s has astounded the European apparel industry, Australian-born Hodge is a good advertisement for his book. Just two years ago, frustrated with the lack of results from his semi-regular gym workouts, he approached Rowland-Smith, an Australia-based trainer of elite athletes, and asked him to help develop an effective and time-efficient fitness program. Says Hodge: "I simply asked Rob to take a program he'd use for an elite athlete and modify it for my needs. I work hard, I travel a lot, I socialise and drink, I get stressed and I'm nudging 50. On the other hand, I don't want to break world records, I just want to meet my own expectations in fitness."

If Hodge was the Fit For Business "lab rat", then Rob Rowland-Smith was every inch its "guru". The "Sandhill Warrior", as he is known to his squads of professional athletes, business people and rehabilitation clients, is a brilliant trainer and motivator. Since his career beginnings as physical education master at The Kings School in Parramatta, west of Sydney, he has served a mix of clients from champions to couch potatoes, adapting the training techniques for the former to motivate the latter.

Over the past 20 years Rowland Smith has condition-trained premiership-winning football teams and world champion surfers. But while he takes great pride in the successes of his champions, he is no less thrilled to see one of his stockbroker clients fulfill his fitness potential.

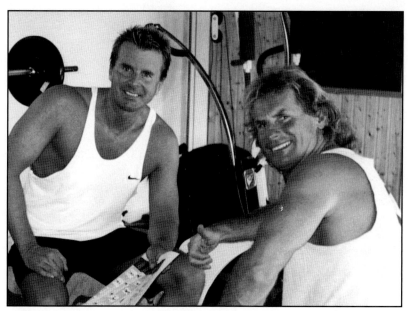

Hodge and Rowland-Smith at work on FFB, Bidart, France, July 1999.

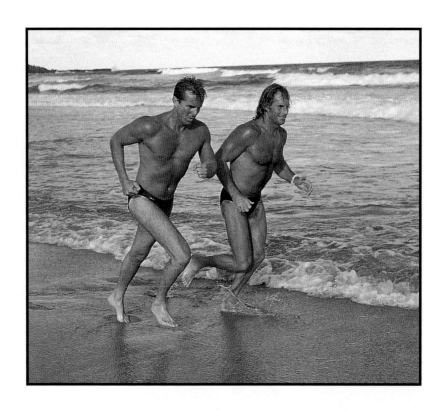

Contents

FFB

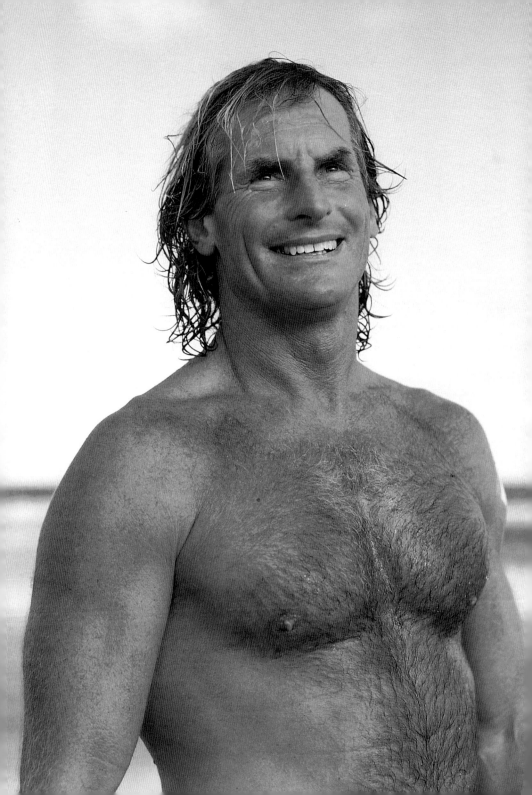

Introduction

Rob Rowland-Smith

I've always felt uneasy taking orders, unless I knew a bit about the background and the motivation of the person issuing them. Since I'm going to be your personal trainer in FFB, in a sense I'll be issuing the orders, so let me try to tell you where I've been and where I'm coming from.

Physical fitness has always been my life. Enjoying sport and physical recreation as a kid, and then doing very well at it as a young man, I realised that physical preparation was the key to good performance. But, beyond that, it just made me feel really good. I felt it gave me an edge that the other guys didn't have.

From a very early age I enjoyed the satisfaction of feeling healthy and good about myself. I learned to enjoy the soulfulness of working alone, of running along a beach with nothing but the wind in my face and the salt air in my lungs. Physical fitness became my passion, then my obsession!

So when I left school I worked for a few years at a variety of jobs - lifeguard, landscape gardener, even as a nine to five briefcase bandit. I wanted to experience all these things before I committed myself to studying, because in the back of my mind I had this plan that if I educated myself in physical education I could pursue a career that enabled me to live the active life I craved. It was going to be a hard road, so I figured I owed it to myself to work out if there was an easier way. Who knows, I might have been happy as a lifeguard all my life!

Ultimately I went to university and teachers college and I did really well. I just loved physical education, still do. Can't get enough of it, whether it's attending seminars or just reading. I got a degree in physical education and a diploma of teaching. I specialised in sport psychology.

In my last year at university I applied for and got a job at The Kings School, Parramatta, and it was at that stage that I became involved in fitness conditioning. I was still very much a competitive sportsman, involved in rugby, the new sport of triathlon, and of course I surfed, although my new job out in Sydney's inland suburbs cut down my time in the waves.

At Kings I settled into an extremely satisfying tenure that was to last 21 years. I not only ran the phys ed department, I helped coach the rowers to five Head Of The Rivers in a row, I was coach of the rugby First XV and a housemaster as well. The school went through a very successful period in sporting achievement, and it felt great to contribute to that success.

Around the same time I started at Kings I got a contract with Western Suburbs Rugby League Club, the quintessential "battlers" of the league. I was friendly with dual international Steve Knight and I used to drive out to training with him and have a run with the boys. Their coach, Don Parrish, said to me one night: "Rob, we really like your approach, why don't you join the coaching staff next season?"

At that stage, the mid-1970s, the concept of fitness conditioning was very new to rugby league. In fact I was one of the first fitness conditioners to be signed to a rugby league club. At Wests back then the club ethos was dominated by its skipper Tommy Raudonikis and his crew. These hardbitten guys trained really hard, but they lived hard too. There was quite a contrast between the exclusive Kings School by day and rough as guts Lidcombe Oval at night! But the three years I had at Wests was the best grounding I could ever have had. The players were aware of fitness conditioning but not in a sophisticated way. I believe the key to fitness conditioning is being able to relay your message. You have to be able to get through, to communicate, and my time at Wests certainly taught me that.

And we had immediate success. Our first game of the season was against Jack Gibson's Eastern Suburbs, who'd thrashed St George 38-0 in the

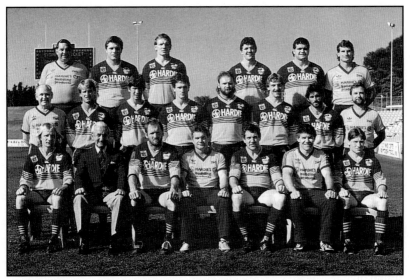

Parramatta's Premiership-winning side in 1986. Rob far right in the back row.

previous year's grand final. We were the battlers, but we went out first game, with the benefit of pre-season conditioning, and we beat them. It was a great start to the season and we did very well after that.

After my three seasons at Wests I took a break from football for a while, then went to the Parramatta club, where I stayed for 14 years. They were vintage years too. We won several premierships and we had a lot of fun. The players were gifted athletes and they had a great attitude to training. In fact, several of them still train with me today.

Over those years working at Kings and with elite rugby league players, my training methods were constantly changing, being refined. I've always had a thirst for knowledge, and whatever I'd learn, I'd apply to my programs. During the Parramatta years I started doing a radio fitness program on Sydney's 2UE, then a spot on Network Ten's Eyewitness News, and finally I graduated to the speaking circuit, linking my knowledge of health and fitness to motivation and self esteem issues.

Then, in the mid-80s, my first marriage broke up and, in reaction to the trauma of that, I moved back to my roots on Sydney's northern beaches. Even though it meant long hours commuting, it was the best thing I could have done, because it put me back in touch with the beach.

I started developing my own training programs on the sand, and that led to quite a few personal training clients. One day at Palm Beach I was approached by Wendy Botha, the South African born surfing world champion who'd become an Australian citizen and made her home in Sydney. Wendy had won her first world title as a South African, and she'd just won her second as an Australian. She was extremely proud of that, but she was also in a bad way, physically and psychologically. She was recovering from knee reconstruction surgery that was in danger of putting an end to her competitive career.

Wendy had been watching me training on the sand and she came hobbling over and asked if she could train with me. I jumped at the challenge because I knew it would take me down a completely different road. You don't train a surfer the same way you train a footballer. In rugby league you need a good base of endurance, as you do in surfing; you also need power and speed in both. But how you get there is totally different.

A rugby league player goes straight up and down the field, hitting that line of defence, so he needs to develop speed and explosive power. He needs anaerobic training with long recovery periods. Short sprint work and plymetrics get him out of the blocks quickly, and low repetitions of heavy weights give him that power to propel forward.

A surfer is essentially a gymnast on water. He needs an endurance base for paddling and for hold-downs in big surf, and he needs power in his legs to drive the surfboard in tight arcs. In the upper body he needs the muscle definition of an athlete but no extra weight to push around.

The absolutely essential differences in preparation I first noticed when I developed a program for Wendy Botha have become the key elements in my approach to fitness conditioning for individuals, and now in the Fit For Business programs. Basically, it's horses for courses.

My work with Wendy led me to another former world surfing champion, Martin Potter. "Pottz", as he is known, was also born in South Africa and relocated in Australia. He had won his world title in 1989 and was widely regarded as the most exciting and explosive surfer on the tour or off it! But since his title win he'd let his mind take a little holiday. He needed a new focus, new motivation. We trained through a summer, then he went to Victoria for the Bells Beach Classic and was

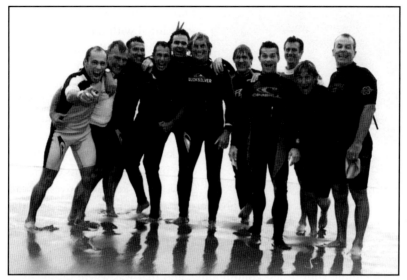

A winter workout at Palm Beach. Tom Carroll is on the left.

beaten in the final by a Californian journeyman. We had a lot of work to do, and suddenly Pottz realised it and we got started on what turned out to be a successful liaison.

For me, working with Pottz provided another valuable lesson in my ongoing education - the importance of psychological preparation in all our training programs, whether we're seeking a world title or simply the motivation to get out of bed in the dark and do it!

From Pottz my path through surfing's elite took me to Tom Carroll, twice world champion in the early '80s, and still on the professional tour when we got together nearly a decade later. Tom was turning 30 and about to step down from the rigours of the pro tour, but he still wanted to be able to accept the wildcard entries offered to him and be able to perform at the top of his ability, so we started working on a program which would carry him through the next decade.

I have no hesitation in saying that Tom is the best and most dedicated athlete I've worked with in any sport. He is still an elite athlete, and surfing as well as he did when he was world champion as he approaches 40. There is a lot of my experience with Tom in this book, just as there is some of the learning I've acquired in my work with hundreds of people.

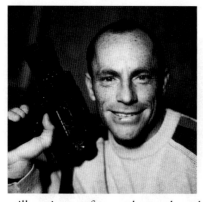

Through Tom Carroll I became acquainted with the executive staff of Quiksilver, the international surfwear corporation which for many years has been the biggest player in the $US2.5 billion surf industry. Founded by a couple of Australian surfers 30 years ago, Quiksilver has never lost touch with its roots, despite its enormous growth. Its key executives are all still active surfers and snowboarders in their middle years, and the corporate philosophy was very much geared towards protection of lifestyle, for the executive staff as much as the pro staff! As you get older, you can't expect to have an active lifestyle unless you work at maintaining your fitness conditioning, and that was where I came in.

One of my first missions on Quiksilver's executive floor was to develop a program for the CEO of Quiksilver International, Bruce Raymond. A former professional surfer, Bruce had a hereditary disposition towards heart problems and he was battling with his weight and the stress of constant travel to oversee the company's international operations. We started out just trying to get him back into shape, but he became so focussed that he ended up doing a full triathlon! Now, in his middle 40s, Bruce is still surfing very big waves and enjoying life to the utmost.

By 1994 I was working with most of Quiksilver's elite surfers as well as a core group of executives. I had long service leave due at Kings, so I began taking the third term off and travelling to Europe and then on to Hawaii with the professional surfers as they headed towards the business end of their tour, with immense pressures on them to retain or improve their all-important world rankings. By 1996 this had become almost a full-time job and, with great sadness, I resigned from The Kings School. On my trips to Europe I began working out with Harry Hodge, the Australian-born head of Quiksilver Europe. As Harry and I trained in his home gym in the hills of Bidart in the beautiful Basque country of south-western France, we began to jot down ideas for a specialised program for...well, for people like Harry. He was 47 and had no

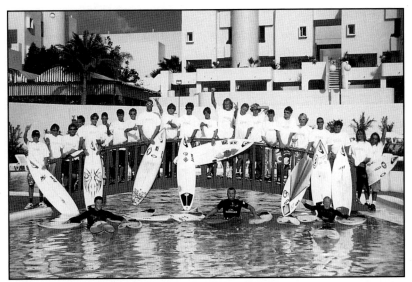

Quiksilver surf camp in the Canary Islands, 1999.

aspirations to be an elite athlete. He simply wanted to retain a level of fitness in which he could take personal pride, and which enabled him to enjoy his strenuous work and travel, his young family and his sports - snowboarding and surfing.

Harry had been working out by himself in the home gym for a couple of years, but frequently he'd become disheartened by his apparent lack of progress. He was a busy guy and often he seemed to be putting in long hours for little reward. When this happened in business, he immediately questioned the process, so that was what he did with me.

Harry's problem was basically that his workouts weren't addressing his specific needs. They weren't doing him any harm, and it was all great stuff if you happen to be a gym junkie - not if you've got another life.

I soon discovered that, like me, Harry Hodge studied the lessons of every one of his life experiences, and as our workouts took shape he extracted every minute detail from me. "Why are we doing this? Will there be any less benefit if we just do this?"

For many months we worked out daily, scribbled notes between super sets, refined our programs until we had what I believe is the most time-effective, directed and no-nonsense fitness program available today. The

proof is in the results already achieved, and for me there can be no greater incentive to go on developing FFB than to step onto a plane and walk through the business class section. There I'll see dozens and dozens of Harry Hodges; men and women who have reached the pinnacles of their careers through the hard work and driving ambition that's written in their eyes. They deserve to derive maximum personal benefit from their best years by being as fit and healthy as their schedules will allow...and most of them don't realise how fit that can be.
Until now.

Rob Rowland-Smith
Newport Beach, Australia
October 1999

Introduction

Harry Hodge

Since I was a young boy I've always been involved in some sort of sporting or athletic activity. In childhood it was football, cricket, swimming or running; from my 20s through to my late 40s it has been tennis, golf, surfing, snowboarding or working out in a gym. Although I've had my moments I've never really excelled at any of these sports, but I guess it's fair to say that when we started Fit For Business I had a good base to start from.

However, at three different times of my life I've been out of shape and generally unhealthy. On each of these occasions I've been struggling with my business and career. Now this may have been pure coincidence, but with hindsight as my ally I would say that, in the majority of cases, health, fitness and success seem to go hand in hand. A healthy person is a happy person, and fitness breeds efficiency.

In my early 20s I worked as a journalist with one of Australia's leading newspapers. It didn't take me long to subscribe to the then-accepted and time-honoured work ethic of the morning newspaper hack. This meant drinking at lunchtime before actually starting work, enjoying a few more beers over the dinner break while at work, then having a few more "with the boys" after work.

It wasn't too long before I came to enjoy the drinking more than the work, and it was time to look for a new direction.

In the late 1970s I ran a film production company which was in serious trouble. Again I found myself "excessing" rather than exercising, finding solace in everything but the important things. Anyone who has felt the full weight of a company's declining performance will know that pressure in business is like air pressure in a tyre - if you release the valve for too long, everything goes flat. That's what happened to me. Paradoxically, while my approach to business had gone flat, excessive living had caused my body to balloon, at least in my terms, from 160lbs to 180lbs.

Again I had to seek a new direction. I moved to a quiet country town on the east coast of Australia, became a vegetarian and adopted a clean and healthy lifestyle. By 1982 I was back in great shape and planned a move to Europe to start an exciting new licence of the Quiksilver surfwear company. It was an extremely challenging move involving language and cultural difficulties and unknown market factors, but I wasn't daunted in the least. I felt as fit in body and mind as I had ever been.

But by 1986 the pendulum had swung and I was in trouble again. Ironically it was the success, rather than the failure of the new business which created the problem. A longstanding personal relationship had just ended, and the growth of the business required immense commitment of time and effort in order to manage it. Work became my entire focus, resulting in way too many late nights of "stress relief" at the local bar. Again, I got out of shape very quickly.

Luckily I met the woman who is now my wife and the mother of our three beautiful children, and my lifestyle turned around overnight. But at 37 I found it was much harder to get back into shape than it had been at 21, and I realised that if I was going to stay fit through my middle years, I would have to commit myself to a consistent personal fitness program.

Accordingly, since about 1987 I've been fairly active in fitness programs, but I noticed that the pounds still didn't come off as easily as I thought they should. And my business life continued to take me around the world with too many plane rides, too many social events and too many featureless hotel rooms. My constant travel interfered with every fitness program I undertook, but at least I was doing something. Or so I would tell myself as I watched my body thicken.

Opposite page: Harry in the French Alps, 1998.

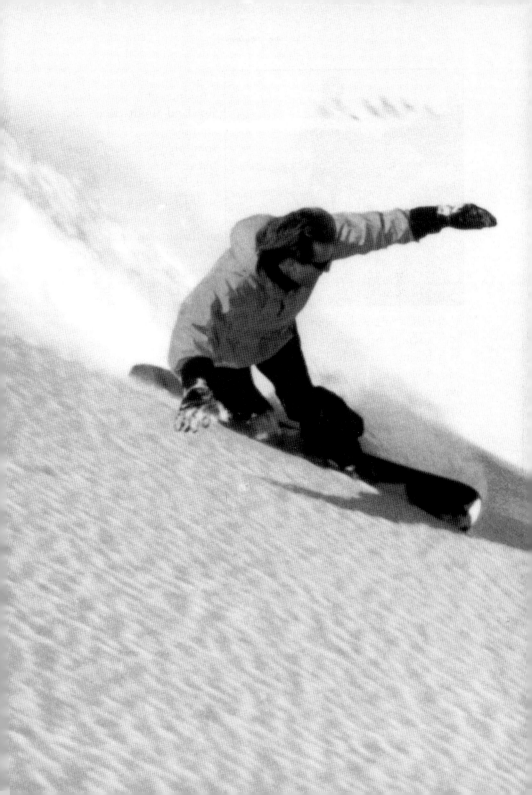

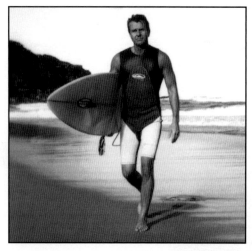

Then in 1996 I started working out with Rob Rowland-Smith, who was training Quiksilver-sponsored athletes. From my very first conversations with Rob I realised that the stuff I was doing to stay in shape was fundamentally inefficient, using up too much time for too little result. For example, when I worked with weights I was unknowingly preparing myself for a future as a front row forward, rather than creating the upper body strength necessary for a middle-aged executive.

As a businessman I had long been interested in time-efficiency, so I started working with Rob on an all-round fitness program for people like myself - cash rich but time poor. Every non-essential item had to be stripped away, we had to determine what kind of program would provide maximum benefit for minimum outlay. It wasn't easy designing Fit For Business; nor is FFB this year's three minute miracle cure. It requires the kind of discipline and dedication that got you where you are today, but that's all it requires.

I turn 50 in the first year of the new millennium and I am probably in the best shape of my life. I am in charge of a very successful company, have a great family and a financial security that makes life very enjoyable. Again, I ponder the correlation between health and fitness and business success, but there are many other reasons for taking your own health and fitness seriously.

I read recently: "The greatest gift you can give to your family is your good health." But a gift is something you chose to give. I would take it a little further, and say that maintaining health and fitness is an obligation you have to your family.

I'm not a fitness fanatic. I have learnt, like most people, that a good balance in life is the key to happiness. How often have you heard the expression "health, wealth and happiness"? Always in that order. I'm proud of the fact that I'm able to provide a certain amount of security for my family, but what I hold more highly is that I am now doing everything I can to ensure I stay healthy and fit so that I can experience and enjoy my children's growing.

One of the reasons I believe I have been successful in my profession is that I have always ensured that whenever possible I give myself a competitive edge. Let me give you an example. In 1984 when we started our company in France we had a turnover of approximately $US1 million. In 1998, as a subsidiary of a public company, our sales in Europe topped $US100 million. Clearly a growth curve like that requires an equal and complementary growth in management skills. I realised quite early on that I would have to strive constantly to improve my skills at business if I was to remain at the helm of the company.

I began to read and listen to everything I could about business and self improvement. There is a lot of garbage in the marketplace, of course, and no one should blindly embrace any of these programs. But there are also a great many beneficial books and programs. The ones that worked for me were Tony Robbins' Personal Power, a 30-day self improvement program, and Stephen Covey's best-selling The Seven Habits of Highly Effective People. I carry copies of both these programs with me at all times. They have become part of my road map for life.

But, having worked my way through just about every business book available, I can tell you that there is one element to business success that is constantly overlooked. And that is health and fitness.

The days of the stereotypical businessperson being overweight, overworked and over-stressed are well and truly gone. Today we live in a society that celebrates health and fitness. And yet in many of the world's major businesses, middle and upper managers still pay very little attention to their personal health and fitness.

Just recently I liquidated my entire share portfolio (not that large, I admit) because I felt that as an investor I was being denied essential information concerning the companies in which I had invested. Although I had access to profit and loss and balance sheets, sales, gross profit, expenses and even inventory levels, I had no way of knowing if the managers of those companies were fit and healthy.

Since I, like most managers, regard people as a company's greatest asset, I found it extraordinary that I could not get a personal balance sheet on the people who ran the companies.

So I sold up!

If you think I over-reacted, consider this. Fortune Magazine published the sad tale of Robert Gouizieta, the former CEO of Coca Cola and one of the leading business figures of the 20th century. Mr Gouizieta died still in the prime of his career. A 60-a-day smoker, he had apparently refused company medical examinations for several years.

To me, this is like over-valuing inventory or propping up accounts receivable. If Mr Gouizieta wanted to kill himself with nicotine, that's his business, but when he hid the state of his health it became the business of his shareholders.

Our Fit For Business program is designed to not only keep you fit and healthy through the busiest and most important years of your career; it is designed to make you more effective in everything that you do. I hope that it becomes as much a part of your working life as your commitment to your company's balance sheet.

Harry Hodge
Bidart, France
October 1999

Chapter 1

What is FFB ?

Rob Rowland-Smith

After Harry Hodge and I had worked out together for a few months, I began to see more clearly what he wanted out of a fitness program, and we worked together to create it. We were enjoying the work so much that our gym sessions sometimes stretched more than two hours.

One day Harry sat down on the bench, took a long swig of his water bottle and said to me: "This is great but I haven't got the time to do this every day. What you have to do is get me the benefits and compress them into an hour-long session I can do, say, five times a week, because that's all I've got."

That was a challenge, but it was really the birth of those aspects that make Fit For Business unique. Basically the tapered-down program encompassed, in the course of just one hour, all the different aspects of fitness training I'd been developing over 20 years. It was a cross training program which encompassed work on cardio-vascular, strength, flexibility and muscle endurance. Our major consideration was that, like Harry, the people who would most benefit from the program had very little time to allocate to it, so we worked on getting everything into a one hour session, just five times a week.

Our aim was to make Fit For Business the most time-efficient fitness program in existence. Ironically, many people who are successful in business are very good time managers, except in one area. When it comes to physical fitness, they plead that they haven't got time. Well, of course they have the time for FFB. They just have to realise that you have to make time for fitness, just as you make time to read marketing reports and production statistics. Our program requires a time investment of just five hours a week. That's 3% of your time.

Time allocation pie chart

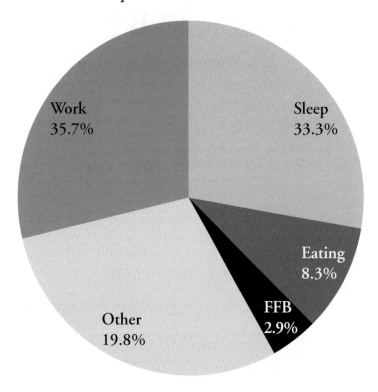

Long before I started working out with Harry Hodge I began a group training session for businessmen in Sydney's Domain Park. It was a three-times-a-week session that we called "Pain In The Domain". Because we were in a park rather than a gym, we didn't have access to weight training facilities, but in every other way it was a cross training session like FFB. We'd run, stop, do a set of upper body exercises, run again...I've always believed in cross training as the most efficient means of achieving fitness, simply because I don't believe that any one exercise can make you fit. For example, if you run and do nothing else, your legs will be in great shape but your upper body will be getting no work at all. It's a very good cardio-vascular workout, but you have to spend an enormous amount of time running to get the benefits.

Anyway, what I noticed in the Pain In The Domain sessions was that the variety in cross training not only gave the entire body a good workout, it gave my businessmen friends a lot of fun. Whereas they might have been bored running or swimming for an hour, in cross training they were constantly being confronted with new challenges, and they loved it.

Since cross training is the foundation on which FFB has been built, I should take a few moments to fully explain it. Cross training is a circuit-style workout that works all muscle groups, using only basic equipment but embracing all components of physical fitness. It combines:

- Aerobic fitness
- Muscle endurance
- Strength
- Power
- Flexibility
- Speed
- Agility.

Cross training is a non-stop workout that can raise the heart rate to gain maximum benefit but still be controlled; it is a workout that can tone and shape muscles, improve flexibility, increase strength and develop stamina. With the right guidance, a cross training program offers people the opportunity to exercise at their own level but still make gains. It is a workout that is both fun and self-fulfilling.

Let's look in more detail at each component of physical fitness covered in our FFB cross training program.

Aerobic fitness

Or circular-respiratory capacity. This means the ability to persist in strenuous tasks for long periods of time. The limit of persistence is determined primarily by the functional capacity of the cardio-respiratory system, ie heart, lungs and blood vessels.

Muscle endurance

This is the capacity to persist in localised muscular effort for long periods. The correlation between aerobic fitness and muscle endurance is really the cornerstone of physical fitness. These two components, when combined, form the plank upon which FFB's commitment to maximum benefit from minimum time is built.

Strength

The measure of strength is the maximum amount of force that a muscle can exert. While bodybuilding programs are structured around increasing those maximums, FFB's emphasis is on functional capacity rather than pretty pecs. Strength is a biproduct of our program.

Power

This is simply strength with another factor added - speed of contraction. Again, the development of power is a biproduct of FFB.

Flexibility

The functional capacity of muscles and joints to work through a full and normal range of movements.

Speed

The ability to move quickly. While it is not a requisite for optimal health and fitness, it is also another helpful biproduct of FFB.

Agility

Generally defined as the ability to change direction quickly and effectively while moving.

The warriors of ancient Greece and Rome were very fit men because they had to be. Their culture decreed that it was most definitely survival of the fittest, so they trained every day, practising with their weapons, running in full armour, doing the things they would have to do well in battle or die.

Fit For Business is not designed to make you a warrior, but I have read widely about warrior cultures because I am intrigued by the way in which fitness was achieved by simple repetition of the things they had to do in the line of work. Today it often seems to me that we've made fitness too sophisticated, too inaccessible. You have to have the right gym equipment, the right clothes and so on. In creating FFB, we've taken a couple of steps backward towards those ancient civilisations. You need to buy virtually nothing, and you can do the program anywhere, anytime. (You can even do it in your armour!)

Later in this book we'll be discussing ways and means of getting you motivated to do this program, but it's interesting to note that the task of simplifying FFB is one of the things that has motivated me for years. In fact we need to go back more than a decade, to a time when it was customary for Parramatta rugby league first team to go out to Parkleigh Prison a couple of times a season and play touch footie with the inmates. We're not talking prison farm here. Parkleigh is a maximum security prison and our boys were mostly lifers. As we played, guards patrolled the walls armed with Armalite rifles.

Despite the rather oppressive atmosphere, we found those games highly enjoyable, and I was quite receptive when the superintendent asked me to come out on a regular basis and run what he called a "fitness rehabilitation program".That's what it was - rehab - and my team of tough, rough guys had no motivation to do mine or any other program, except that it might be marginally more interesting than pacing the quadrangle.

I started going to the prison once a fortnight for a two-hour training session. Believe me, Parkleigh was somewhat different from what I'd been used to at the Kings School, Parramatta. At my day job I had all the equipment money could buy, and a bunch of kids who regarded phys ed as the highlight of their week. At the prison I had a 50-metre field, a chin-up bar, two medicine balls and a bunch of thugs with attitude.

The situation really brought me back to basics. I had to deal psychologically with the hardest group of people imaginable in a facility with zero equipment. It was a great experience for me because it took me back to the grass roots. I had to rethink my methodology to make it work in this situation, and the sessions left me emotionally and physically drained. But I still believe that without that experience I would never have been able to pare back our programs to absolute basics. And there were other rewards too.

A few years after the Parkleigh sessions had stopped, I was in a pub in

Parramatta after a pre-season training session. A fellow across the bar kept looking at me and I thought there was something familiar about the face. Eventually he made his way over, introduced himself in a shy way and warmly shook my hand. He said he'd been part of my group at Parkleigh and that after I'd stopped coming some of the men had continued the sessions by themselves, using the notes on the workouts I'd left them.

He said: "Fitness has turned my life around, mate. I started to look at myself in a new light. I started to keep check on my progress in the fitness program, and soon I was using the same techniques to check my progress in life. And I haven't looked back. I got sent to a minimum security farm and then I got paroled. I've got a job, I've gone back to school at night and I feel like I'm in control of my life for the first time. I just want to thank you for getting me started."

I walked out of that pub feeling ten feet tall.

Are you fit enough to start FFB?

We strongly recommend that anyone over the age of 35 take a full medical examination before starting FFB. The Human Performance Laboratory at the Sydney Academy of Sport uses the following questionnaire to identify people who need further medical screening before beginning a fitness program. If you answer yes to any of these questions, you must not start FFB without a full medical.

- Has a doctor ever told you that you have heart trouble?
- Do you frequently get pains in your heart or chest region?
- Do you often feel faint or have severe dizzy spells.
- Do you often feel excessively short of breath on exercise?
- Have you ever been told that your blood pressure is too high or has it been recommended that you take medication to lower your blood pressure?
- Have you ever had a blood test for your cholesterol level which reported that your cholesterol was too high?
- Are you or have you been a regular smoker?
- Are you currently physically inactive (less than two hours of exercise per week)?
- Have you ever suffered a stroke?
- Has any close blood relative ever suffered a heart attack or stroke before the age of 70?
- Do you have any bone or joint problems such as arthritis, or any old sporting, motor vehicle or work injury that you think may be made worse if you exercise?
- Have you ever suffered heat stroke or any other heat-related illness?
- Have you any personal or family history of diabetes or epilepsy?
- Is there any other medical or health reason which would prevent you from increasing your physical activity?
- Do you take any medication or drugs which may affect you during an exercise program?
- Are you allergic to anything?

The basic equipment

For an outlay of $600-900 in Australia (£250-300 in the UK), you will have all the necessary equipment for FFB. How does that compare with city gym or golf club membership? We visited three good suppliers in Sydney and one in London to compare prices.

Chatswood Exercise Equipment

1. Infinity brand bench with rack and leg extension (home gym quality)	$199
2. Bar (5'6")	$49.95
Bar (6'0")	$59.95
3. Weight plates per kilo	$2.50
4 x 10 kg	
2 x 15 kg	
4 x 5 kg	
4 x 2.5 kg 100 kg total	$250
4. Dumbell handles	$80
(set of 4 x .5kg and 4 x 1.5kg plates)	
Total	**$638.90**

Once Only Fitness, Dee Why

1. Own brand bench with rack and leg extension (commercial quality)	$524
2. Bar (5'6")	$45
Bar (6'0")	$55
3. Weight plates 100kg at $1.80	$180
4. Dumbell handles (small)	$40
(large)	$45
Total	**$889**

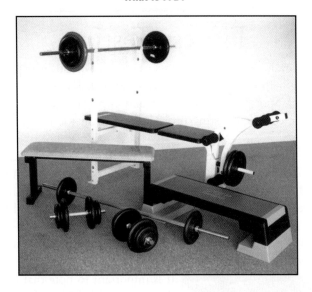

Sampson's of Rydalmere

1. Own brand bench with rack and leg extension $335
   (commercial quality)
2. Bar (5'6") $40
     Bar (6'0") $45
3. Weight plates 100 kg at $1.50 $150
4. Dumbell handles (small) $30
                (large) $35

Total   **$635**

UK Mail Order

1. Bench press with rack and leg extension   (£100) $250
2. Barbell x 2   (£30) $75
3. Dumbell x 2   (£20) $50
4. Weight plates 100kg   (£120) $300

Total   (£270) **$675**

Fitness Testing

In order to evaluate the effectiveness of our Fit For Business programs we enlisted the help of the Human Performance Laboratory at the Sydney Academy of Sport. Christine Grice and her team put the FFB team through the complete testing procedures used in the evaluation of elite athletes.

The three people tested were of similar age but at very different levels of fitness. Rob Rowland-Smith is a fitness professional for whom training is a way of life and a livelihood. Harry Hodge is a businessman who has been working out with the FFB programs for 18 months. Phil Jarratt is a publisher and marketing consultant who has dabbled with FFB during the course of putting together this book, but at the time of testing he had not worked out at all for several months.

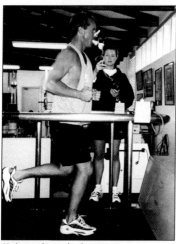

Hodge tests his aerobic fitness.

It is important to note that none of the three men tested were "unfit". Hodge and Rowland-Smith were FFB-fit, Jarratt had a reasonable residual fitness level as a result of regular surfing and beach jogging.

The results were very interesting. Jarratt's aerobic fitness was slightly above average for his age group (again thanks to the jogging). Hodge's aerobic fitness was well above average, prompting Christine Grice to exclaim: "I can't believe he gets those results without running."

How 18 months of FFB has worked on Harry Hodge

December 1997	May 1999	Results
Weight: 78kg	Weight: 80.3kg	Lost 4kg of body fat
Body fat: 23% (18kg)	Body fat: 17.9% (14kg)	Lost 1 inch from waist
Chest: 41 inches	Chest: 44 inches	Gained 6kg of lean muscle mass
Waist: 34 inches	Waist 33 inches	Gained 3 inches in chest

Phil Jarratt: age 48, height 174.2cm, weight 73.9kg, body fat (skinfolds) 15.1%
Harry Hodge: age 49, height 181.6cm, weight 80.3kg, body fat 17.9%
Rob Rowland-Smith: age 47, height 182.2cm, weight 88.3kg, body fat 12.7%

	Phil Jarratt, age 48	Harry Hodge, age 49	Rob Rowland-Smith, age 47	Age Av
Upper body strength				
Bench pull	65kg	70kg	91kg	N/A
Bench press	57kg *	85kg	119kg	N/A
Abdominal strength	1	4	4	2
Lower body power				
**Vertical jump	22 (30)	44 (40)	45 (40)	N/A
Anaerobic capacity				
Peak power	8.1	11.5	11.0	10.0
Total work	192.3	258.0	261.8	250.0
Lactate	10.7	11.7	11.1	10.0
Aerobic capacity				
***Max. heart rate	177	183	201	N/A
VO2 max (ml/kg/min)	40.14	44.0	60.0	37.0

* Jarratt was restricted in this test due to a rotator cuff injury.
** The figure in brackets is the expected result, based on height, weight and age.
*** The spread between resting and maximum heart rate is a very good indicator of cardiovascular fitness. For example, Hodge has a resting heart rate of 55 beats per minute, a normal working day rate of 65, and a maximum of 183. A sedentary person of similar age might have a heart rate spread of 80 to 140, less than half Hodges. This means that the heart of the second man is only being asked to do half the work.

Chapter 2

A Foundation for Health and Fitness

Firstly, a warning: there are people out there who are going to knock Fit For Business. Some of them may even be educated in the principles of physical fitness, some of them may be personal trainers or coaches. And they will tell you to be wary of our programs. Why? Well, there is always going to be a great deal of subjectivity in fitness training. It goes with the territory. But in the main, the people who criticise FFB will do so because of a basic failure to understand its aims and objectives. It's a little like the company that sets out to be number two in the market and coast, with greater profitability, in the slipstream of the market leader. That company is likely to be criticised by industry professionals for failing to realise its potential. Likewise, FFB is likely to be criticised by fitness professionals because it doesn't adhere to the principles of weight training.

The reason for this is simple. FFB is not weight training. It is not body-building. People will tell you that training with weights on consecutive days is wrong, and it is wrong - if you are training to build muscle mass or size. To achieve these goals you need to "hurt" or genuinely fatigue the muscles at each training session, and then give them time to rest and grow.

FFB is not about this process. FFB uses free weights or body weight as tools of resistance training in an advanced form of cross or circuit training. Cross training can be comprised of any number of activities or exercises that suit you. In FFB we have selected exercises that complement each other, provide variety and stimulate all groups of muscles. If you use the program properly, you will not "over-train" and thus avoid injury. FFB is designed specifically as a foundation for health and fitness in the segment of the population that needs it most. Us.

When we talk about "us", let's make no bones about it. FFB will not suit everyone. It will not suit the career couch potato, nor will it suit the businessman who has taken early retirement to concentrate on competing in 12 triathlons a year. But it will suit anyone who has known a reasonable level of fitness and wants to retain or regain it, and is prepared to put the same level of commitment into health and fitness as he or she has put into building a career.

FFB is specifically designed to provide the most complete all round workout in the most efficient time frame. And efficient is the operative word here. Like most successful businesses, FFB is built on simple logic. No tricks or gimmicks, no miracles, no shortcuts. We ask you for a commitment of five hours a week (we'll take three, but we're asking five and four will be a bonus) and the return on your investment is a level of fitness that will improve every aspect of your life, both personal and professional. The effects of the program will be felt almost immediately, but the real value of the FFB approach is that its basis of efficiency and time management applied to exercise will stay with you forever.

Enough about what FFB isn't. Let's look at what it is and how its theories are applied.

Fit For Business is, over and above everything else, a great cardio-vascular workout. The heart is the most important muscle of the body, a large muscle that requires continuous movement, and this is one of the major considerations of any cross training program. In FFB we move from exercise to exercise, maintaining a high pulse rate, working aerobically, or literally, "with oxygen". This means that the muscles are working continuously, and that the heart and lungs are forced to keep up the supply of blood, oxygen and nutrients. At the same time, working aerobically throughout the session increases the body's ability to store energy-producing glycogen in muscle cells.

The basic premise of FFB is that we get you "in the zone" and keep you there for between 40 minutes and an hour. The zone is that mysterious place where you are deriving maximum cardiovascular benefit and burning the most fat at the same time. Exactly where the zone is varies between individual metabolisms, but the simplest and best equation is to start with a heart rate of 220 beats per minute, subtract your age, then take 70-80% of the remainder. For example, if you are 49 years old, the equation is 220 - 49 x 80% = 136.8. This figure represents the high end of the training zone. A normal heart rate at rest for a 49-year-old would be around 70, so you will feel the exertion, but not to the point where you cannot talk or watch TV or appreciate your workout music. However, getting in the zone requires effort and concentration, and if you are able to conduct a conversation throughout your workout, you're probably not in the zone.

Recently at a gym in Hawaii we noticed a girl come in and go straight to the step machine with a bunch of magazines which she proceeded to flip through while she stepped very slowly. Then her mobile phone rang and she had a 15-minute conversation while reading and stepping. She should have been at the hairdressers! Of course, any exercise is better than none, but if you want FFB to work for you, you have to take it more seriously than that.

The 70-80% equation also applies to the weights you use in FFB. For example, if you can comfortably lift 10 kg for a set of repetitions, start out lifting eight. Women doing FFB will most likely be using lighter weights than men, and in order to stay in the zone, they should perform more repetitions.

Now, let's examine in greater detail how FFB will improve fitness.

Cardiovascular

Undoubtedly the strongest muscle (by weight and size) in your body is your heart. The figures bear this out. It beats 2.5 billion times in an average lifetime, sending five quarts of blood to every cell of the body every minute, which adds up to 220 million quarts in a lifetime. It is an amazingly efficient muscle, but like all muscles, it will become weak and even atrophy with neglect, whereas with constant exercise, it will perform more efficiently and actually grow in size and strength. Aerobic exercise oxygenates the blood, allowing the heart to beat stronger and slower, achieving more with each beat.

FFB Training Zone (Men and Women)

Age	Low (bpm)	High (bpm)	Age	Low (bpm)	High (bpm)
35	130	150	51	114	134
36	129	149	52	113	133
37	128	148	53	112	132
38	127	147	54	111	131
39	126	146	55	110	130
40	125	145	56	109	129
41	124	144	57	108	128
42	123	143	58	107	127
43	122	142	59	106	126
44	121	141	60	105	125
45	120	140	61	104	124
46	119	139	62	103	123
47	118	138	63	102	122
48	117	137	64	101	121
49	116	136	65	100	120
50	115	135			

The FFB Training Zone Chart is the recommended level for training. The low end equates to approximately 70% of your maximum heart rate and the high end equates to 80%. We recommend that beginners start training no lower than the low end threshold, and work towards the high end as quickly as possible.

Advanced FFB users (more than a year on the program) can up the level to 90% to increase gains.

Strength

How often do you hear, "I don't want muscles, I just want to be fit." As we get older, our bone density decreases, particularly in women. Our bones become brittle, our body shapes change and we become subject to diseases like arthritis and osteoporosis. The best way to combat this deterioration is through gaining strength. Being strong means that your muscles are able to work continuously for much longer. Being strong also means that your immune system is stronger. Being strong increases your abilitiy to deal with stress without experiencing fatigue.

Muscles are like armour plating. They support your frame and they protect your internal organs. Our skeletal systems simply would not work if we didn't have muscles, and the stronger the muscles are, the better they will work. Human movement involves the interaction of 200 bones and at least 650 muscles. One step requires the exertion of 200 muscles, the lifting of one leg at least 40. Obviously muscle tone leads to more efficient working of the entire body. So often, elite athletes forget this simple and basic tenet of fitness. They neglect their strength training, become thin and weak and start to suffer illness because their immune systems are not working properly.

Muscle atrophy is the shrinking of muscle due to lack of exercise. If an active person is laid up for a lengthy period, their muscles may atrophy as much as 20%. If they continue not to exercise, the muscle turns to body fat. Old people often have twinges when they perform simple activities they've done all their lives, which is a direct result of not using those muscles often enough. If you let your car sit for a while, the engine will seize up. It's the same thing.

Flexibility

The more exercise you do, the more you increase the range of muscle movements, thereby creating greater flexibility. In FFB, the exercises are designed to use all the muscle groups in fast repetition, which builds strength and increases flexibility at the same time. But it is absolutely vital that you stretch before and after exercise to avoid muscle strain.

In fact, if you've been sedentary for quite some time, or if you've gradually tapered off your exercising in recent years, there are three rules

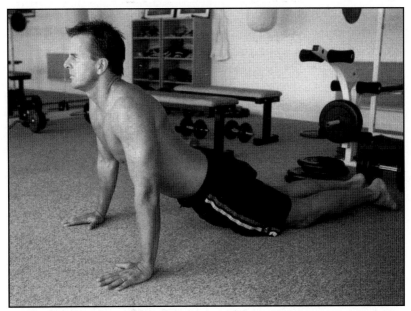

Stretching after an abs workout.

you must apply to FFB:

1. Always, always stretch before and after.
2. Warm up slowly. Spend as much time as you can afford getting the blood flowing.
3. Use good form and technique. This takes time and attention, but it will give you better results with less risk of injury.

The gimmicks

Over the past 20 years we've seen a never-ending stream of "quick-fix" fitness programs, videos and equipment trotted out and flogged to death on the shopping channels. Some of these have a sound physiological basis, but it's a pretty good bet that the more extravagant the claims, the less likely they are to be true. And there are thousands upon thousands of ab machines and the like gathering dust in garages and attics.

We're not going to waste your time by detailing every fraudulent advertising claim in the health and fitness industry, but one recent gimmick is worthy of comment - "electromyostimulation", which many of you will be familiar with from visits to the chiropractor or physiotherapist. The electrode stimulation of muscles is used with great efficiency in the treatment of sports injuries, but muscle stimulation as a form of fitness training got a pretty bad press when it emerged as a technique used by Eastern Bloc athletes about a decade ago. This hasn't stopped several companies from coming out with carefully-worded advertising campaigns designed to convince you that you can "plug in" and get fit.

You can't. A "fitness" device that doesn't stimulate the cardiovascular system is simply not a fitness device.

In tandem with the gimmicks are the misconceptions about fitness training which seem to have increased exponentially in line with the rapid rise of a fitness culture over the past 20 years. This is most evident when you visit a city or hotel gym and see people doing training routines that serve no purpose and, in some cases, could be doing them harm. How often have we seen people walk into a gym and, without warming up, go straight to the bench press. One set later they're onto the stationary bike for 10 minutes, the step machine for five, then 100 rapid-fire sit-ups with a towel around the back of their heads!

There are so many legitimate approaches you can take to fitness training, and so much bogus advice as well, that it is understandable there is confusion. Giselle Droguett, an instructor at Sydney's Temple of the Body and Soul, blames "simplistic regimes" promoted in magazines for much of the confusion. She told a newspaper reporter: "The latest thing I've heard is you only need 30 minutes of exercise a week to lose weight. That's really only health maintenance...but you would never read that in a magazine."

The point is that all fitness programs that work are based on sound principles which you need to understand before you start. Fit For Business is no exception, which is why it is imperative you read these chapters. It always helps to know the destination before you begin the journey, but in this case it is vital.

Five common myths about fitness training

1. **I can't lift weights because I bulk up too much.**
   You will only bulk up if you lift extremely heavy weights and do four to five sets of repetitions with long recovery periods. For all-round fitness you must do some form of resistance training.

2. **Women shouldn't lift weights.**
   Women can use light weights and high repetitions to tone and shape. The popular "pump" classes are a form of weight training.

3. **You should never lift weights and do aerobics together.**
   Only if you're doing pure strength training or body building. For fitness and conditioning plus greater cardiovascular benefit, combine the two.

4. **When lifting weights you should always have recovery time between sets.**
   Again, only if you are strength training and building muscle mass.

5. **You only need three 20 minute aerobic sessions a week to get fit.**
   A myth promoted by magazines selling quick fixes.

Chapter 3

Motivation

Feeling good
Rob

What motivates me is feeling good. It's as simple as that. I want to feel good all the time, and two things in my life can achieve that for me. The first is my own level of fitness. When I'm fit I'm happy. The second is what every trainer or teacher worth his salt feels, and that's the joy of seeing other people fulfill their potential.

In my view there is no greater motivator than feeling good. Everyone I've ever trained successfully has been motivated by the desire to improve themselves in some way so they can feel good about themselves and life in general. It doesn't matter whether you're an elite athlete or an overweight, stressed out, middle-aged executive, the name of the game is the same. It's about maximising your potential, and to do that you have to believe in yourself.

In Fit For Business the goals that we've set are all attainable, provided you have the motivation to do the work required. If you've bought this book, you're already on the way! You've been motivated by what it promises, but it doesn't promise anything unless you can build on that motivation. Consider this little book as a challenge. It doesn't take very long to read and at the end of it, you'll have a very good idea of what is required of you to meet that challenge. Of course you could then put it

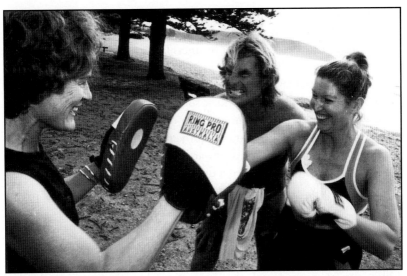

Boxing mit workout on the beach.

up on your bookshelf and never look at it again, but that is highly unlikely, given that you were motivated enough to buy it in the first place. However, just as there are plenty of dens, garages and attics full of discarded fitness "toys", there are many bookshelves stacked with self-help tomes read once and forgotten. That's a case of the "help" being there but the "self" lacking the motivation to get on with it. Don't let this happen with FFB or I'll jump out of the pages and rip your bloody arms off!

Seriously, what we've found with FFB is that once people begin the program, their motivation becomes greater as they progress. In that it's quite different from sessions with a personal trainer. In my experience a lot of people find these stimulating and different for a while, then less so, and then they stop making the appointments. They find it too hard to stay motivated, and they blame the PT for that. And maybe there's something in it, maybe he's driving too hard, or not hard enough.

We don't give you that luxury with FFB. If you read the book, if you understand why we're going to be doing what we're doing, if you take in the big picture as well as the nuts and bolts of how to do the program (and it's pretty simple), then you've got no one to blame but yourself if you drop out before you've accomplished your mission.

No one to blame but yourself. Sounds pretty tough, doesn't it? Well, the point is that you are in control of this program and the way you use it. No one else, just you. As in your business life, you are the master of your own destiny with FFB. And, also as in your business life, you know that gains are gains. Achieving 50% of budget is not great, but it's way better than 30%. You might have to kick some butt, but you're not going to close down the division on the strength of one lousy performance.

It's the same with FFB. If you fall off the program, regard it as a fall, not a plunge into the abyss. And beware the rationale that I've heard so many times: "Yeah, well, I tried a fitness program but I was just too busy to do it regularly, I wasn't getting anywhere and I realised I'm just gonna have to live in the body I've got."

In a word, bullshit! Anyone who's basically healthy can benefit from FFB no matter how busy they are. Better time management is just one of the things you'll learn through doing it. All it takes is getting started. Once you've experienced the immediate benefits you'll feel your motivation growing until working out is just part of your life, it's a joy, not a chore, and you miss it when you don't do it.

Motivation is really just a simple rewards system. If you don't get a reward in reasonable time, your motivation goes away. With FFB the long term rewards are very substantial indeed - better physique, stronger, healthier constitution, better attitude to work and play, and more energy to enjoy both. The short term rewards are undoubtedly more subtle, but they are nonetheless tangible and recordable. The better you record your early progress, the less likely you are to lose your motivation. And, as most of you probably know, there are few greater feelings in life than that real joy of accomplishment, of knowing you have done something positive about your fitness.

Getting started
Harry

The hardest thing for me was getting started. A cliche I know, but it's true. The fact that I'd been working on inefficient programs for a while didn't help - I'm a businessman, I like to see results and I hadn't seen any. I felt I'd been making an investment and getting no return.

FFB didn't give me instant results either, but the logic of the program was so clear that I could work towards my goals without feeling disheartened, and once I'd pushed through "the wall", everything started to change. The results were evident not just in my fitness level but in my approach to work, family life and relaxation too. I had a vague notion that a better level of fitness would increase my ability to handle stress, but I didn't properly appreciate the fact that FFB would actually make me function better as a businessman. It has, and that began from the day I decided that I was going to make room in my schedule to do the program, even if it meant making some sacrifices. But in fact no sacrifices have been necessary. Through making space in my life for FFB, I've become a better time manager. I don't try to cram my day like I used to. Instead I adopt the approach I use in FFB, methodically working through my agenda, taking time out to reflect and review my progress.

I'm actually fitter today at almost 50 than I was at 21, and I'm a better businessman because of it!

The Big Five-O

Speaking of the Big Five-O, I guess it's a time of life when a lot of us begin to wonder what old age will hold. I remember as a teenager, and even into my 20s and 30s, just dismissing old age as something that could never happen to us - we were forever young! Then suddenly you look at your expected life span and you realise that time is running out. You're on the downside of middle age, the long, slow slide to the grave has begun.

So why do I feel in such good shape? Why do I feel better, physically, emotionally, intellectually, than I have at any previous time of my life? Have I discovered the fountain of youth?

Imagine, if you will, a shopping channel (or even a major chat show) and I'm on it and I'm telling you I've discovered the fountain of youth, that here is something that will ensure you live longer and have fun until you're ancient, that it's virtually free, that's there's no limit on supply and that the success ratio is staggering. I can feel the free call switchboard lighting up like a Christmas tree.

All of the above is, of course, true. The fountain of youth is called exercise, and there's only one small catch. We have to be motivated and have self discipline to use it.

Recently a close friend gave me a great book called "Growing Old Is For Sissies". It's a bunch of photos and profiles on people from their 60s through to their 90s who are fit and healthy and enjoying life - sometimes in fairly bizarre and eccentric ways! I found it totally inspiring because, as new medical research is now telling us, age doesn't have to mean slowing down.

A study undertaken at the American College of Sports Medicine indicated that older people had no problem adapting to quite rigorous exercise programs and responded particularly well to strength and endurance training. The study found that men and women aged between 55 and 75 "significantly reduced a number of functional declines associated with aging" through a well-balanced fitness program. Strength training helped offset the loss in muscle mass and strength, while endurance training improved most aspects of cardiovascular function. Chuck in improved bone health and a reduction in the risk of osteoporosis, better posture and greater flexibility, and you've got a fairly convincing argument for keeping up with exercise. It's a case of "use it or lose it".

The rocking chair test

Personal Power author Anthony Robbins has his "rocking chair test", which I believe is one of the simplest and most effective personal mantras of motivation. To apply the test, you just close your eyes and imagine yourself at an advanced age, sitting in a rocking chair looking back on your life. What would you change? What would you have done better? It's amazing how, seen from this perspective, so much of what we do in our lives seems like needless clutter.

It's a line from an old gag, but it's also very true: few of us will reach our deathbeds and say, "Gee, I wish I'd spent more time at the office."

Likewise, I'm prepared to bet that the guy on the table about to have open heart surgery after a lifetime of sedentary behaviour would sign a blank cheque if you told him, "I can get you out of this mess if you agree to exercise just five hours a week."

Health tests for the over 50s

I'm looking forward to turning 50 in the new millennium. I see it as the beginning of an enjoyable and challenging phase of my life, but I also know that I'm reaching an age when my personal responsibilities to my body are increasing.

I've been doing this stuff since I turned 40. If you're 50 or close and you haven't been having regular medical check-ups, don't leave it any longer. It takes an hour out of my schedule once or twice a year, which is a lot less time than you devote to keeping your car running smoothly.

These are the basic medical tests I suggest:
- cardiogram once a year
- blood pressure check twice a year
- blood sampling for cholesterol, sugar, urine once a year
- PSA blood sampling for prostate cancer
- skin cancer checks once a year, twice a year if you live in a warm climate
- breast examination and pap smear for women once a year

In addition to these tests performed by my doctor, I also use some of my own tests. I'm not obsessive about it, I'm not a hypochondriac. I simply take the view that the more knowledge you can gather about your own body, the more effective you can have it running. I monitor my heart rate almost every time I work out, I check my under-arms and testicles for lumps while showering, and most importantly, I regularly check the results of my bowel movements. Not a terribly pleasant subject, I admit, but the fact is our stools are good indicators of the health of the bowel, the largest and one of the most important organs in the body.

Healthy stools don't float, they are two to three inches long, in one piece and range in colour from light brown to brown. Black or red colour indicates internal bleeding and should be checked out immediately. Grey indicates a surplus of fat in your diet. A grey stool will probably float. HH

Confidence

The message is clear: we have to take control of our lives while we can. It's not easy, but it's totally achievable and all it requires is your motivation and your self discipline. And that gets down to your confidence.

My favourite sporting heroes are Michael Jordon, Muhammad Ali and Don Bradman, three brilliant athletes with very little in common other than their absolute confidence in themselves. Confidence is what gave them the winning edge, and it is purely a mindset. Optimism is simply confidence applied to a particular set of circumstances. It's something for which I'm sometimes criticised by my business associates when I make broad-based statements about goals we are going to achieve. But I welcome the criticism because it becomes my competitive edge. It makes me even more determined to meet the goals I've set.

The negative work cycle

One of my business associates (not necessarily one of the above who dares to criticise!) is an extremely competent operator. He is tall, good looking, popular, confident and secure in his job. Only one flaw will stop his rise to the top. He doesn't take his health and fitness level seriously enough.

At the moment I'm trying to encourage him to take up the FFB program, and he does train with me intermittently, but more often than not he cites his workload as his excuse to skip training. Just like I used to. Hopefully in time he will realise that you actually have to develop the discipline to walk away from the workplace and do some exercise. You will come back in better shape and work more productively.

My friend is locked into a negative work cycle. Work drives his personality and the cycle goes like this:

- Too much work
- no time to exercise
- overwork
- stress
- health problems
- inability to perform at work
- too much work.

Why? Well, he should be intelligent enough to work it out but there's an element of ego here too. Because he's so good at his work, he's much more comfortable in that environment than in a training environment, and something is telling him he should stick to his own beat. I can understand that, and it's why FFB, which he can do in total privacy if he wishes, will be so good for him. But will he stick with it? I hope so, because if he doesn't his health and fitness will begin to jeopardise the thing he holds most dear - his career.

The mirror test

There are infinite ways to check your progress in a fitness program, but I prefer the simplest, and it's not the bathroom scales. Nine times out of 10 they'll give you entirely inaccurate information anyway. Throw them out, the same way you'd throw out office equipment that gave you wrong information.

The best way to monitor your progress is to look in the mirror. Strip off and take a long, hard look at yourself. Get a second opinion from your partner. A second opinion is always good, and if you feel any kind of embarrassment about doing something to help yourself, this will help dispel it. Make a list of the stuff you see and don't like, so that you can prioritise those areas once you start the program. If you've got a spare tyre you can't stand, for example, work harder on your abs until you've got it back under control.

Judy's story
Rob

Prior to 27 January 1997, my wife Judy was a world champion athlete, holding age records for 800 and 1500 metres on the track, and having represented Australia in triathlon. She was in her late 40s, super fit, highly-competitive, hard-driven.

Then, on that day she was forced into the back of a truck while doing her cycling training, breaking her neck and suffering severe trauma of the spinal column, a broken jaw and severe facial and head injuries.

The first verdict was that she would be a paraplegic, but after a spinal fusion this was changed to quadriplegic. She was told she would have partial use of her right arm, very limited use of her left and that she would be extremely lucky to walk again. She went straight into rehab and after months of hard work and sheer determination, she can now run at 65% of her former ability. She can ride a bike on grass and ultimately will reach about 70% of her former all-round athletic ability. I sat with her in hospital when the doctors gave her that terrible prognosis, and she's disproved them. They told her she'd never compete again and she's going to disprove that too. Why? Because she had a background of tremendous athletic discipline, and she had a body that was fit and strong enough to survive her accident, an impact that would have killed most women.

So if ever I'm lacking motivation I don't have to look very far. The best inspiration an athlete could have is right here at home.

Boothy's story

I met Jeff Booth a few years back in Hawaii after he'd been signed by Quiksilver. He was a young professional surfer from Laguna Beach in California, rated number 33 in the world at the time, but he had a few problems so we brought him back to Australia to go to work on him. Now I can cite rugby league premier teams and surfing world champions and many other elite athletes I've worked with who've gone on to do brilliantly, but Boothy's story gives me the greatest satisfaction because it's about someone with plenty of natural ability but plagued with injuries and self doubts. It's about how you can turn that around through sheer force of will.

Back in Australia we sat down to draw up some attainable goals for him. I said, "Where do you want to finish this season?" He said, "I'd like to improve on 33."

I turned on him: "Bullshit, that's not a goal. Top 10, that's a goal!" Boothy shook his head and said he didn't know about that, self doubt, self doubt. I told him he could, and he would.

Over the summer, with the pro tour in recess, I worked him like a slave. We had group training sessions three times a week and he started to really fire. At the end of each session we'd have one of my "ironman" races, which might consist of a 100 metre run, 100 metre swim, then another 100 metre run to finish. It was a highly competitive group and

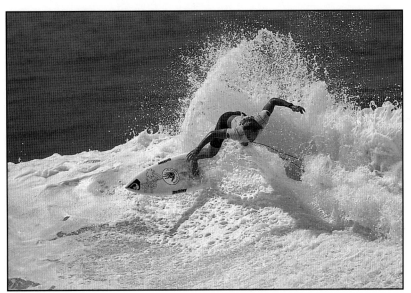

Jeff Booth competing at Hossegor, France.

this was a good way to finish with them really amped up. I bought a yellow Speedo swim cap and had "No 1" printed on the front and "Catch me if you can" printed on the back. Okay, pretty silly, I admit. Just one of those dumb things you do to motivate a group. Anyway, they got off on it. The winner of the ironman on Monday would get to wear the cap on Wednesday, and so on. The guy who won the most got to keep the cap at the end of the season. Guess what? It was Boothy.

Let's jump ahead a few months to France, midway through the pro surfing tour. Boothy's doing quite well, ranked about seventh or eighth and he's through to the quarter finals in the Rip Curl Pro at Hossegor. I run a training session each evening for the Quiksilver competitors, just a short workout, some stretches, a jog then a bodysurf or a game of touch footie. The evening before his quarter final Boothy dives full stretch on the sand for a try...and jars his neck. It was an old injury aggravated, but he couldn't move it. I sat up with him most of the night. Ice, stretch, ice, stretch. But it was no better in the morning.

I found him on the physio's bench in the competitors tent half an hour before he was due to hit the water. He grimaced and said: "It's no good, Rob, I can't move my head. I'll have to pull out."

I was prepared for this. "Fuck you!" I boomed. The physio took a hurried step backwards. I pulled the yellow cap out of my pocket and dangled it in his face. "What does this mean to you?"

He said: "It means a lot of hard work on the sand."

"And did you have to hurt a bit to win it?"

Boothy tried to nod his head and I noticed there were tears streaming down his face, but I kept it up. "Well you're going to hurt today too..."

Before I finished he was up off the bench and pulling on his wetsuit.

He won his quarter final, beat world champion Kelly Slater in his semi and was just beaten by Rob Machado in the final. The whole event was agony for him, but Boothy forced the pain into a room by itself and locked the door on it while he got on with the job. He finished the tour that year as number 6 and improved to number 4 the following year.

People using FFB won't have to endure Boothy-style agony, but whenever I think about his effort that day it makes me train a little harder. Maybe it'll do the same for you.

The Motivation Quiz

1. Do you set goals for yourself?
a) rarely or never
b) sometimes
c) always

2. If someone criticises your performance do you
a) tend to take offence
b) ignore them
c) take note of it and possibly apply

3. If you've had a very late night and you have an early morning appointment, do you
a) cancel it
b) make it, just
c) get up an hour earlier, work out to clear the head, then make it

4. If you have a work deadline that is going to be difficult to meet, do you
a) ask for an extension
b) panic
c) work harder and longer

5. What do you think when you look in the mirror?
a) we are what we are
b) I can fix this next summer
c) I will fix this now

6. How do you rate your quality of life?
a) low
b) medium
c) high

7. How do you spend your relaxation time?
a) don't have any
b) doing nothing
c) doing the things I enjoy

8. How often do you exercise?
a) intermittently or never
b) occasionally
c) regularly

9. How do you rate your sex life?
a) not great
b) okay
c) great

10. How do you think people perceive your physical presence?
a) bit of a wreck
b) not too bad for age
c) fit and healthy

Score one point for every a) answer, two points for every b) and three points for every c).

10-15: Well, you're very honest, which we appreciate. You probably have a self-deprecating sense of humour and aren't as bad as you make out, but it does appear you are going to have to work very hard to make FFB work for you. And, as long as you keep that sense of humour going, you'll do it.

15-20: The bottom end of this range is a bit of a worry - the not quite couch potatoes - but 17 up you'll be okay, as long as you're prepared to work hard and change a few perceptions.

20-25: You are our people, motivated enough to want to change, and needing to.

25-30: You're probably already working on a fitness program. Don't worry, FFB is better.

Chapter 4

Nutrition

Rob

You can't have an effective fitness training program without an effective diet. It is absolutely essential that the body is refuelled adequately to give you the energy to perform the program and regenerate.

But there are, of course, 101 ways of looking at nutrition and how to achieve a nutritious diet. I'm not a nutritionist so I tend to soak up information from every source offered and then use my commonsense filter to offload all the rubbish and come up with what works best for me. I never dictate what to eat to the people I train, but I do preach my own little gospel in three parts:

1. Regardless of your current eating habits, start eating a solid, healthy breakfast.
2. Learn how to achieve balance in your diet.
3. Practice moderation.

In an ideal world we would all eat about five small meals a day, rather than three big ones. This keeps your metabolic rate high, enabling you to burn more calories. When I'm training all day this is exactly what I do. If you're working in an office, it's a little trickier. You can't be forever

Rob's week

Monday
Breakfast: cereal, baked beans on toast, two muffins with jam, fruit smoothie.
Snack: apple.
Lunch: ham salad sandwiches and two pieces of fruit, cup of tea.
Dinner: grilled chicken fillets with salad, bread rolls, fruit and ice cream, plenty of water.

Tuesday
Breakfast: meusli bars and fruit between training clients, cup of tea.
Lunch: ham, cheese and avocado sandwiches, two pieces of fruit.
Dinner: actually a late supper after training finishes at 9pm - lasagne with salad, bread rolls, two pieces of fruit, water.

Wednesday
Breakfast: cereal, eggs and pancakes, fruit juice.
Lunch: mixed sandwiches, fruit, water.
Dinner: steak, vegetables, salad, fruit platter, water.

Thursday
Breakfast: meusli bars and fruit, water.
Lunch: mixed sandwiches, fruit,water.

excusing yourself from meetings to knock off a snack! However we can all adhere to the general principles of eating light and eating right.

In my experience by far the worst dietary habit in businessfolk is their approach to breakfast. Whether it's because they're just too busy to grab more than a cup of coffee (which might provide a short-lived kickstart but has no nutritional value whatsoever), or because they're obsessed with the idiot logic of "exercise is good, eating is bad", the vast majority of executives I know start the day the wrong way. I am constantly amazed at the number of people who show up for their morning workout without having had any breakfast. They don't wake up thinking, okay, I've fasted for eight hours, the meal I had last night has been used up in regenerating muscle tissue, my digestive processes are working better now than at any other time of day, better build an energy

Dinner: (very late again) beef stirfry with vegetables and noodles, bread rolls, fruit, water.

Friday
Breakfast: muesli bars, date scones, fruit, water.
Lunch: home-made vegetable soup, biscuits with avocado and cheese, fruit, cup of tea.
Dinner: home-made hamburgers, potato chips, green salad, fruit and ice cream, water.

Saturday
Breakfast: porridge, baked beans on toast, fruit smoothie.
Lunch: chicken, avocado, cheese and lettuce sandwich, water.
Dinner: Thai chicken curry with rice, bread rolls, fruit and ice cream, two beers.

Sunday
Breakfast: cereal with banana, cup of tea.
Snack: fruit and meusli bars.
Lunch: pie and finger buns, water.
Dinner: barbecued fish, potatoes, green salad, fruit, one beer.

reserve for the day ahead. No, they tend to think that skipping breakfast is a relatively painless way to cut back, a lot easier, say, than skipping the networking lunch.

Life is far too short to spend time stressing over exactly what's in every meal that's put in front of us. However, a basic understanding of what constitutes a balanced diet is important, and simple enough. If you're an active person, you need quite a lot of carbohydrate, fibre and protein, plus enough fat to cover what you're burning. The less active you are, the less fat you burn and the less you need. If you look at my diet and Harry's over an average week you'll see that there are considerable differences. I need more bulk, he has more social pressures affecting his intake of rich food and alcohol which he has to balance the rest of the week. But the similarity between the two is that they're mostly just

Harry's Week

Monday
Breakfast: cereal (Fruit & Fibre), one banana, cup of tea.
Lunch: mixed sandwiches, quiche, half a brownie, one banana, orange juice.
Dinner: cashew nuts, grilled chicken, salad, mixed fruit, water.

Tuesday
Breakfast: cereal (Fruit & Fibre) with banana, toast and Vegemite, cup of tea.
Snack: apple.
Lunch: ham, cheese and tomato sandwich, cup of tea.
Dinner: fois gras on toast, sole meuniere, salad, three beers, three glasses of white wine.

Wednesday
Breakfast: cereal (Fruit & Fibre), toast, orange juice.
Lunch: vege burger and salad sandwich, cup of tea.
Dinner: chicken sausages (2), chicken and salad, fruit, water.

Thursday
Breakfast: cereal (Fruit & Fibre) with strawberries, toast, water.
Snack: apple.

ordinary meals. No denial, no extremism. Balance and commonsense. Which brings me to my third gospel, moderation. Almost all of the athletes I work with will go overboard on occasion, maybe celebrating a victory, maybe commiserating over a loss. Whatever, that's fine as long as you are prepared to discipline yourself when it matters. The guy who trains with me at midday, then goes out and has the four course lunch from hell, washed down with a few bottles of wine and a couple of cleansing ales, well, he's not fooling anybody. He may as well not bother training that day. The food will sit in his stomach digesting very slowly, causing drowsiness and general discomfort. He'll go home feeling bloated and unfit. But the people who regard food intake as an integral part of training simply don't do that. They time their run and they time their fun, if you like.

Lunch: ham, salad, avocado sandwich, cup of tea.
Dinner: tomato salad, magret de canard, potatoes, two beers, three red wines.

Friday
Breakfast: cereal (Fruit & Fibre), banana, water.
Lunch: club sandwich (no bacon), tea.
Cocktails: four beers.
Dinner: mixed salad, lamb chops, three red wines.

Saturday
Breakfast: two fried eggs on toast with cheese, cup of tea.
Lunch: McDonald's with the kids, chicken burger, fries and orange juice.
Snack: apple.
Dinner: corn chips with salsa and avocado, barbecued chicken with salad, three beers, three red wines.

Sunday
Breakfast: one egg, two slices of toast, cup of tea.
Snack: toast and Vegemite.
Lunch: chicken salad, two beers, four white wines.
Dinner: grilled chicken, salad, water.

Harry

If you're serious about fitness you have to be disciplined about what you eat, especially when you travel a lot, leaving your normal routines behind. So often while travelling on business I've seen colleagues compensate for the strangeness of their surroundings (or perhaps their nerves about the business to be done) by gorging themselves on food and wine. Usually they are totally oblivious to the ingredients of the dishes presented, and often take a macho delight in their ability to devour what's offered. ("I've got guts of iron, nothing they eat over here can hurt me!")

While I admire their zealous commitment to the advance of multi-culturalism, I tread carefully when I travel, even on familiar beats. It's not that I don't enjoy discovering new and interesting food - far from it.

It's simply that experience has taught me that there are so many occasions on the road when you cannot control your food intake, you have to utilise those occasions when you can.

For example, I do a lot of business in London so I try to stay at the same hotel where I know the restaurant and I know the room service menu backwards. Here it's very easy for me to be sociable or to kick back in my room without wondering what's in the strogonoff sauce.

When I travel I often carry Australian nutritionist Rosemary Stanton's "Fat & Fibre Counter" in my briefcase. This little gem is about the size of a hip pocket note pad and is a very handy reference guide to those most important aspects of nutrition. Which is not to say it addresses the whole argument. It doesn't. There are saturated fats, polyunsaturated fats and mono-unsaturated fats, and while there is not much to say in favour of saturated fats, the body does need fatty acids from the other two. The Fat & Fibre Counter only lists the fat content of each food once, although it does carry a warning asterisk on foods in which saturated fat makes up more than a third of the total fat content.

Basically I stay away from the asterisks as much as possible (a McDonald's Big Mac has 27 grams of fat and more than 10 of them saturated) and use the fat and fibre count as a guide to foods I'm not sure about. I aim for at least 40 grams of fibre a day and no more than 40 fat, and as much of that as possible mono-saturated. For example, one avocado would give me my whole fat quota for the day (40g) and so would a piece of Kentucky Fried Chicken and a medium serving of french fries. The difference is that the avocado is "good fats" while the junk food is almost entirely saturated "bad fats". I'm not obsessive about fat and fibre counting (and I don't even think about calories), but after a restaurant dinner I may refer to the book and make a quick tally. If I find I've gone way over my limit, I'll make sure I restore the balance by eating light the next day.

At home we eat fresh, simple meals, but I do have a passion for French duck. At least once a week I'll put some lean magret de canard on the barbecue and we'll enjoy it with a fine Bordeaux red. Then there are the occasional Saturday sessions at McDonald's with our young kids. They're growing up bilingual with a broad appreciation of French culture, but they're suckers for a Big Mac like kids the world over. (And, to tell the truth, it's not that much punishment for us either!) And finally, there's my egg habit. I like my eggs for breakfast once or twice a week and, fortunately, the nutritionists are coming around to my way of thinking. The cholesterol panic of a few years back put the humble googie in the sin bin for a while, but the fact is it's high in protein, low in fat and contains vitamins A, D and E. My case rests.

To cover the fact that I enjoy a varied, and sometimes rich diet, I practice under-eating. I

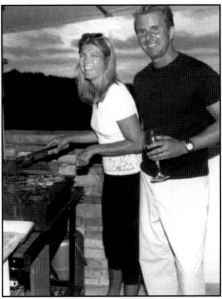
Summer evening barbecue at home in Bidart.

believe that in affluent society almost all of us over-eat. Considering the amount of physical activity we undertake each day, even a "normal" diet is probably too much. Of course, metabolisms vary, but in a great many cases, a 20% reduction in food quantity across the board would have no ill effect. This is largely due to the fact that our "norms" are drawn from another age, when work was much more physical.

This theory was put to the test some time ago. Two groups of monkeys were fed differently over a trial period of 10 years. The first group was fed what was generally considered to be a "normal" diet. The second group was fed 20% less of exactly the same food. At the end of the study it was found that not only did the second group show no ill effects from the smaller quantities, but by almost every index used, the group was healthier than its counterpart.

I try to adhere to the 20% less principle. In a restaurant if my dinner companions are having two courses, I'll skip the first or else have two starters instead of a main. When my wife cooks at home, I never miss out on anything, I simply have smaller portions. Of course, the harder I train, the more I need to eat, and I factor this into the equation by

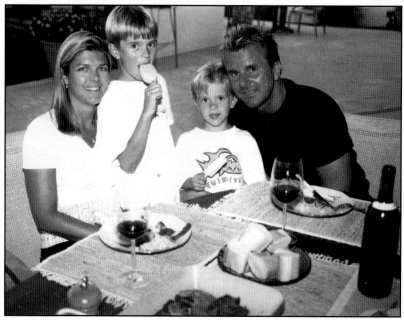

Dinner with Sandee and our boys Mathieu (left) and Tommy.

keeping my training diary up to date.(These days I enjoy training so much that it often comes as a surprise to me that I've worked out seven days straight!)

I also drink wine with dinner most nights of the week. We'll address the issue of alcohol consumption in the next chapter, but in terms of nutrition and healthy eating it's important to note here that whether there is wine on the table or not, there will be plenty of water. I try to drink eight to 10 glasses a day, and one glass of water for every glass of wine over dinner. The effects of dehydration during sporting activity are well documented, but there are many other reasons to keep up the supply of water all day - better endurance, better concentration, better resistance to disease, better chance of weight loss are just a few. And unless you're planning to become an endurance champion and work out for several hours a day, don't worry about the fancy sports drinks either. We all know they taste better, but their main function in fitness is to replace electrolytes used up in marathon exercise sessions, like a triathlon or a four hour session in big surf.

Harry's handy hints on eating right

- Eat regular meals
- Never skip breakfast
- Eat light at night
- When cooking eggs use a non-stick fry pan rather than butter or oil
- On bread get used to spreading the butter half as thick as you normally would
- Avoid deep fried foods in restaurants and hotels
- When eating out skip the starter, or have two starters instead of a main
- Skip dessert regularly, regard it as a treat
- Don't believe the words "Low fat" or "Lite" on food packaging
- Eat red meat sparingly, try skinless chicken as an alternative
- Marinate chicken before barbecuing to give it extra taste without adding heavy sauces
- Strike a balance between meat and fish, and always eat a salad with both
- Eat vegetables regularly
- Go easy on the cheeses (easier said than done, living in France)
- Snack on fruit rather than doughnuts or bagels
- Drink at least eight glasses of water a day
- Vary your diet to keep it interesting, and remember, your body doesn't need as much as you think it does.

Vitamins and other supplements

All the vitamins and minerals we need should come from a balanced healthy diet, but most of us have to make compromises and we need to compensate. I stick to the basics, taking 500 grams of Vitamin C each morning. From time to time I also take a course of ginseng and royal jelly, and if I think I need detoxifying, I'll use Musahi Huan The Dispersion.
HH

I'm a great believer in taking supplements daily. I take a multi-vitamin and anti-oxidant combination which is high in C and E. To maintain my immune system I take Echinacea and horseradish and garlic.
RRS

Sheraton Park Tower
L O N D O N
NIGHT TIME MENU

-To Start With-

Minestrone soup with garlic croutons and parmesan £7.50

Cream of chicken soup £7.50

New Forest wild mushroom soup £7.50

Slices of seasonal melon with Parma ham £13.25

Prawn and avocado served with Marie rose sauce £12.50

Traditional oak smoked Scottish salmon £17.20

Tomato and mozzarella salad with a basil dressing £11.75

Traditional service of caviar "golden oscietra or beluga"- Market Price

-To Follow-

Spaghetti bolognaise served with grated parmesan £13.50

Caesar salad with char-grilled chicken £16.25

Grilled baby chicken, marinated tomato, garlic and lemon juice "taouk style" £21.00

Escalope of Veal Viennoise £21.50

Whole Dover sole Meuniere or grilled £25.00

Above is the night room service menu from the Sheraton Park Tower in London, my hotel of choice when I'm on flying business visits. I often need to work through a light meal in my room before getting an early night in preparation for the next day's meetings, so this menu is very familiar. I've circled a few of my regular selections, avoiding anything in a rich, creamy sauce, deep fried or a huge cut of meat. I often have the slices of melon to start, minus the ham. This is just a personal choice - I don't like the combination. Depending on my mood, I'll then go with the veal or the sole. The Sheraton's Veal Viennoise is a good example of "clean cooking", done using minimal oil. I order it minus the rich sauce. The sole, grilled with no garnish, is invariably excellent and close to fat-free, and the selection of vegetables is lightly cooked, fresh, crisp and healthy. And I usually find myself able to pass on the desserts.
HH

Grilled fillet of Aberdeen Beef £24.00

Grilled English lamb cutlets served with French fries £22.00

Classic fresh ground beef burger served on sesame bread, plain or with cheese garnish with French fries £14.50

Whole lobster with garlic butter or as you like it - Market price

Vegetables

Selection of seasonal vegetables £6.00

French beans £3.90, mangetout £3.90, glazed carrot £3.90

Jacket potato, French fries, sauteed potatoes or new potatoes £3.90

Basmati or saffron rice £4.00

-*To Finish*-

Desserts and Cheeses

Fresh fruit salad and cream £6.80

Sugar coated apple pie with cream or ice cream £6.90

Classic creme caramel £6.50

Cheesecake baked with seasonal berries £6.90

Your choice of ice cream and sorbet £6.90

A plated selection of English and Continental cheeses £9.60

Rosemary Stanton's Fat & Fibre Counter

A few examples from this invaluable little book. Your daily intake of both fat and fibre should be around 35-40 grams. * indicates more than a third of the fat is saturated.

	Fibre	Fat
A medium-sized apple	3.0	0
Half a small avocado	1.0	18.0
Fried bacon and eggs	0	32.0*
Half a can of baked beans	10.5	1.0
Grilled rump steak, with fat	0	33.5*
Grilled rump steak, lean only	0	10.0*
Bran flakes with fruit	7.5	1.5
Big Mac	2.5	27.0*

(Rosemary Stanton's Fat & Fibre Counter is published by Wilkinson Books (61 3 9654 2800)

Chapter 5

Balance

Harry Hodge

Balancing the budget

Nobody would dream of running a business without a balance sheet, a profit and loss accounting. Good businesses always have good cash flow, plenty of reserve and control of inventory. I approach Fit For Business exactly the same way.

I aim for five sessions a week because I want to average three or better. If I achieve an average of 4.2 over a year, then I've exceeded budget and I'm happy. If I aimed for three and achieved less, not only would I not make budget, I would not derive the major benefits the program has to offer. My system takes into account three things:

1. My periodically heavy business schedule.
2. Sickness.
3. Goofing off.

I don't often get sick and I don't often goof off, but each year from my home base in France I make six business trips to the US and two to Australia, as well as countless shorter trips within Europe. Last year I spent 75 nights in hotel rooms. No matter how well you look after yourself, a travelling schedule like that can take its toll, and during the year I succumbed to a stress-induced illness which became a bronchial virus and kept me from working out for almost a month.

The episode taught me a very good lesson - to make time in every day, no matter how tight the schedule, to kick back and relax. It also put a

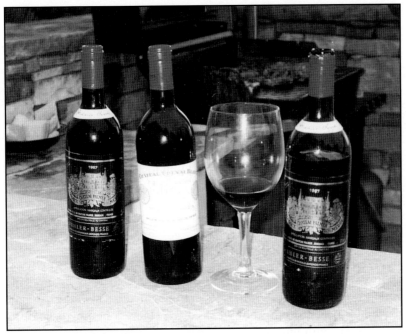

Life is too short to drink bad wine.

dint in my workout average, but because I had quite a few workouts in the bank, I still managed to finish the year with a 4.2 average.

Of course you can't take that much time out of the program and come back and pick it up where you left off, but the efficiency of FFB is such that I was working at about 80% of my previous capacity after one week and back to full strength within two weeks. This would not have been the case with my old workout routines. The reason is that the FFB approach to building strength and endurance is designed to last. The average loss of conditioning is 1:3, which means that it takes three months to lose what you've gained in each month of training. The strength training part of the program is designed to increase your strength by 2.5% per day, but you will only lose it at 1.5% per day you don't work out.

The beauty of this is that for whatever reason you lapse, when you return to the program you are not starting all over again. You pretty much pick up where you left off, and that's a great incentive to get back into the gym. Too often people use a lapse as an ongoing excuse for a lack of self discipline. Oh, I fell off the program so what's the point? Well, the point is that the program is still there waiting for you, and you are already a few rungs up the ladder.

I mentioned goofing off, which might sound flippant but is in fact an essential part of the FFB program. The "money in the bank" theory allows you choice, which any person in business is going to need at some point. For all your best intentions, there will be a time when you have to choose between, say, a networking social function and your promised workout. If you're working on five and building your program on three, you can afford to take the social option without guilt, without feeling you are letting yourself down.

Balancing the lifestyle

In the previous chapter we spoke about the need to take a commonsense approach to the basic dietary principles. While there is no need to embrace any one of the myriad doctrines of diet, in order to gain maximum benefit from FFB, we need to achieve a healthy balance in what we put into our bodies. This principle extends, of course, to the social lubricants which are an everyday part of the business life.

I am a social drinker and I probably drink more than I should. But to me the bottle of Bordeaux Grand Cru over dinner or the Friday evening beers with my staff are non-negotiable items. They are a part of my life that I don't wish to change, and I think my fitness test results verify that I can accommodate this in my overall healthy lifestyle.

The medical evidence on the long-term effects of excessive drinking is irrefutable, but we all know that the medical definition of "excessive" is draconian in the extreme. I don't know any male drinkers who would consume only two standard drinks a day, apart from my co-author Rob, who can only sometimes be coerced to have a cold beer on a hot day. Nor do I know any female drinkers who would regularly stay inside the one-drink-a-day limit. So everyone I know who drinks, drinks excessively by medical standards.

There is also increasing evidence to show that a moderate intake of alcohol is good for you. Researchers at the Kaiser Permanente Medical Centre in Oakland, California found that people who averaged one or two drinks a day were less likely to be hospitalised with heart problems than were teetotalers. Alcohol apparently increases our high density liproprotein (HDL) levels, thus lessening our chances of heart disease through the clogging of arteries. Then there is the French Paradox. The French eat far more dairy products than other Westerners and yet have the lowest rate of heart disease in the Western world. Researchers examined the Gallic diet and came up with the news that we'd been longing to hear - that red wine was Factor X. As it turns out, the French also eat more fruit and vegetables than English, Americans and Australians, but there certainly seems to be an element of truth in the assertion that some alcohol can be good for you.

My personal approach to alcohol is to enjoy it in moderation as part of my daily routine, taking care to miss a day or two a week to replenish the system. I enjoy the camaraderie of end-of-week beers with my staff and feel that this social time together is an absolutely vital part of the company dynamic. I also feel that life is too short to drink bad wine, so I opt for quality over quantity. Overall, I believe I can balance my use of alcohol with my genuine desire to be as fit as I can be.

When it comes to smoking I have an entirely different view. There is no balance between smoking and a healthy lifestyle. You cannot hope to reach anywhere near your fitness potential while you are a smoker. And yet in the '90s we've seen depicted in the glossy magazines a renewed and somewhat trendy association between athleticism and smoking - in this case, smoking cigars.

I get very annoyed when I see photos of movie stars and high profile elite athletes sucking on fat cigars, because I know that the groovy cigar bars of London, New York, Los Angeles and Sydney are full of new wave cigar smokers - fit young people who have been deluded into believing that smoking stogies is cool, that the product of Cuba and the Dominican Republic is somehow exempted from the lethal toxins of ordinary tobacco because the stars use it and it costs a lot of money.

The facts are that cigars have four times the nicotine and up to 40 times the tar of cigarettes, according to the American Health Foundation, so even an occasional Havana will put you into the moderate smoker bracket. In the long term, you need only look at the health warnings on the cigarette packs (cigars sold individually mysteriously escape this indictment) to see the risks you run. In the short term, any kind of smoking has an immediate impact on your ability to fitness train. Says Rob Rowland-Smith: "Smoking inhibits your lung capacity, it inhibits the amount of nutrients absorbed by your blood, and it will damage your heart. If you're a smoker and you don't intend to stop, then you will still derive benefits from FFB, but you won't get anywhere near your potential. I've worked with a lot of smokers and I've seen them struggle with their breathing, particularly in the early stages when you really don't need any discouragement. You want to shake them and say, if you gave away the smokes you'd be so much better! But that's not what FFB is about. It's about adapting a training program to your lifestyle. The rest is up to you."

Balancing the pressure

I've got a really simple approach to business. I write everything down. I have an agenda for everything. Writing down an agenda seems to free up that part of my brain so that it can examine the deeper issues. I don't spend the day grappling with what I'm supposed to do, I attack how I'm going to do it.

For me FFB has the same effect as writing down my agenda. It frees me up for other stuff. It's not so much stress relief as stress prevention, because I'm ensuring that I don't suffer overload. I'm creating my own time and becoming more adept at time management through doing it. I suppose some people could look at my five hours a week and think that, with a young family including three active boys, I was being selfish. I look at it another way. When I come home after a hard day, there are two ways I know I can effectively relieve my stress. I can go straight to the fridge and grab a beer, then give it time to kick in before I talk to the family. Or I can go straight to the gym, work out for an hour and go to my family in a happy, relaxed frame of mind. I know which one my wife prefers, and chances are I won't even need the beer!

A psychologist's report once contended that if every male with a family came home from work and belted a punching bag for 15 minutes before he even acknowledged the wife and kids, domestic violence would be reduced by 75%. I don't know about that but I do know that for the vast majority of people, exercise is an extremely effective form of stress relief.

The stress relief benefits also carry over into your business life in ways that I hadn't expected. I find that when I'm in a regular training pattern, my working day is more ordered and I have more time to devote to the "big picture". And my relaxed approach tends to flow on through the management of our company. We've voluntarily reduced working hours by five hours a week as a result of better performance across the board, everyone is happier and we've provided access to a gym and encouraged all our employees to use it.

In his book "What They Don't Teach You At Harvard Business School", time management guru Mark McCormack says he always gets worried when his employees tell him they're too busy to take a vacation. To him that indicates inefficient leadership, and I tend to agree. McCormack asks his people to work less and accomplish more, and to me that is a cornerstone of good management. The days when we glorified the guy who worked 12 hour days are gone forever.

When I look back at our "hand-to-mouth" days of a decade or so ago, the change of approach today is extraordinary. FFB can't claim credit for all of this, of course, but I sincerely believe that it has helped me focus on the right direction for our company, and the right balance for those who work in it.

On a personal level, while there is no underlying mental or philosophical platform on which FFB is built, I find that I use some of the mental preparation techniques of yoga or tai chi. If I find myself trapped in a hectic business schedule where it seems that skipping an overdue workout would be the path of least resistance, I spend a few moments visualising my workout, the sets, the reps, how hard I would train and the results I'd achieve. Then I visualise what would happen if I dropped off the program for good! I make time for the workout, and I enjoy it all the more for having won that small battle with my own forces of negativity.

Balancing the physique

There are two extreme stereotypes of fitness. The first is the Schwarzenegger model, 350 lbs of rippling flesh and muscle definition with 4% body fat. The second is the champion triathlete or marathon runner, 150 lbs wringing wet and 4% body fat.

Both are extremely fit by their own standards, and both require incredible levels of commitment and dedication. But the bodybuilder almost certainly would not have the cardiovascular capacity nor the flexibility of the triathlete, while the triathlete would not have the strength nor the muscle endurance of the bodybuilder.

Horses for courses, but I don't know anyone who wants to look like either of these extremes, and there is growing evidence that the fitness regime required to reach the top in both disciplines is by no means ideal for long term fitness and health. FFB is a balanced fitness option which combines the best of both these worlds. It is designed to increase strength and muscle endurance without altering body shape, and to give you better cardiovascular performance and greater flexibility without the litheness of a leopard or a greyhound.

Time Management

The best book I've read on stress and how to relieve it is Dr Andrew Goliszek's "60 Second Stress Management"*. Dr Goliszek explains in very simple terms the root causes of stress and offers detailed plans to eliminate these from your life. One of the major causes of stress in a business life is bad time management. Try this quiz from the book, answering the closest option. (1= Always, 2 = Usually, 3 = Sometimes, 4 = Rarely.)

1. I find that I have enough time for myself, to do the things I enjoy doing.
1   2   3   4

2. I write down specific objectives in order to work towards goals.
1   2   3   4

3. I plan and schedule my time on a weekly/monthly basis.
1   2   3   4

4. I make a daily to-do list and refer to it several times a day.
1   2   3   4

5. I set priorities in order of importance and then schedule time around them.
1   2   3   4

6. I'm able to say no when I'm pressed for time.
1   2   3   4

7. I try to delegate responsibility in order to make more time for myself.
1   2   3   4

8. I organise my desk and work area to prevent clutter and confusion.
1   2   3   4

9. My meetings and activities are well organised and efficient.
1   2   3   4

10. I finish one job or task before going on to the next.
1   2   3   4

Scoring key: 10-16 = Excellent time manager
           17-22 = Good time manager
           23-40 = Poor time manager

*60 Second Stress Management, Dr Andrew Goliszek, Bantam Books UK 5.99, Aus $14.95.

Rob's Diary

Monday

6.15am   Bilgola Beach group session for men - sand running, boxing, swimming etc 90 min.

9.30am   Bondi Beach women's group session - sand running, circuit, water work 90 min.

11am   Rope climbing and martial arts session with former SAS soldier client.

12.30pm   "Pain in the Domain" running and cross training session for business people in Sydney CBD. 60mins.

3pm   Paddling session with client, either ocean (Northern Beaches) or still (Pittwater).

4.30pm   Weight session at "Muscle Beach", my outdoor gym at home.

6.30pm   Ironman training with lifesavers from Palm Beach Surf Club. (Summer only.)

Tuesday

6am   Palm Beach sandhill session with client.

7.30am   Bike session with client at Palm Beach.

10.30am   Bondi Beach women's group - higher intensity than Monday.

12.30pm   Low intensity running session with client in Domain.

2.30pm   Paddling and sand-running session with client at Palm Beach.

4.30pm   Rehab weight training at Muscle Beach with injured client.

6.30pm   Rugby training with Manly club.

Wednesday

6.15am   Ironman session at Palm Beach with men's group.

9.30am   Women's group session at Neilsen Park, Vaucluse.

11am   Personal training session - rope climbing and martial arts.

12.30pm   Business group at Boy Charlton Pool, swimming and resistance.

3pm	Paddling session with client at Palm Beach.
5pm	Training with surfers, followed by personal weight session.

Thursday

6am	Palm Beach sandhill session with client.
7.30am	Paddling or walking session with older client.
8.30am	Palm Beach run and weight training session with client.
10am	General fitness with new clients - varies each week.
2pm	Paddling and sandhill running with client.
4.30pm	Rehab weight training at Muscle Beach with injured client.
6.30pm	Manly Rugby Union training.

Friday

6.15am	Ironman training with men's group at Palm Beach.
8am	Bike ride and weights with client.
10.30am	Women's cross training group at Balmoral Beach.
12pm	General fitness with new client.
1.30pm	Afternoon off for personal swimming and weight training.

Saturday

6am	Running session with client at Palm Beach.
9am	Sandhill and boxing session with client at Palm Beach.
10.30am	Walking session with older client, Palm Beach.
2.30pm	Running and swimming session with client, Bilgola Beach.
4pm	Mixed group weight training at Muscle Beach.

Sunday

6am	Paddling session with client, Palm Beach.
8am	Mixed group session in Palm Beach sandhills, hardest session of the week.
11am	Palm Beach Surf Club races in summer.
4.30pm	Rehab weight training with injured client.
6pm	Personal weight training or late surf.

Harry's Diary

Monday
8.30am	Arrive Paris.
10am	Meeting re Champs Elysées shop opening.
11am	Meeting with Peugot management re prototype "Quiksilver 806".
12pm	Review shop set-up, Champs Elyssee.
1pm	Lunch meeting with windsurfer Robby Naish.
2pm	FFB hotel room workout.
4pm	Oversee final preparations for shop opening.
6pm	Shop opening cocktail.
8pm	Inauguration dinner.

Tuesday
8am	Breakfast meeting at hotel.
11am	Depart for Biarritz.
2pm	Meeting with marketing dept re Thursday press conference.
5pm	FFB workout at home.
7pm	Cocktails and dinner at home for international guests.

Wednesday
8am	Preparation for board meeting, home office.
9am	Board meeting.
1pm	Lunch meeting with marketing director.
2pm	General staff meeting.
3pm	Preparation for press conference.
5pm	FFB workout at home.
7pm	Cocktails and dinner at restaurant for overseas guests.

Thursday
9am	Meeting re press conference.
10.30am	Briefing with sponsored athletes Kelly Slater, Robby Naish, Lisa Andersen.
11am	Press conference to launch environmental initiative in Europe.
1pm	Meeting re inauguration of office facility.
2pm	Afternoon off, FFB workout with sponsored athletes.
6pm	Cocktail for our new video release.

Friday

9am	Prepare inauguration speech and run through with translators.
12pm	Supervise auditorium set-up for inauguration.
3pm	Break.
5pm	Final meeting with organising committee.
6pm	Cocktail party.
8pm	Inauguration dinner.

Saturday

10am	Final international meetings.
12pm	Afternoon off with family.
6pm	FFB workout at home.
8pm	Farewell BBQ dinner at home for international guests.

Sunday   Day off with family.

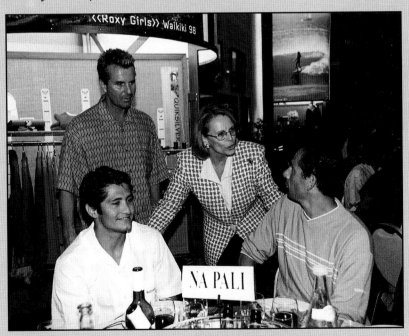

Harry Hodge (back left) with mayor of St Jean De Luz Madame Alliot-Marie and sports stars Bixente Lizarazu and Guy Forget.

Chapter 6

Other Sports

Rob Rowland-Smith

When Harry Hodge made a commitment to the Fit For Business program under my supervision, he had no intention of it becoming his "sport". He already had sports he loved and was quite good at. He felt that FFB would make him better able to enjoy his golf, snowboarding and surfing. As it's turned out, Harry loves working out so much that it has become another sport in his armoury, but FFB's time-efficiency has meant that he still has time for the other things he likes to do.

That's his choice, and as you'll see from the comparitive benefit chart, his fitness level is the winner because no other sport can match the fitness benefits of FFB. As you start the FFB program, you're probably wondering how it will fit into your life alongside your other activities, like your weekly round of golf or Sunday tennis or early morning surf. The answer is that FFB will improve your performance at any sport you care to name. However, the reverse is not necessarily true, and it is important you don't start out thinking that you can interchange your FFB workout with, say, nine holes of golf and think you are achieving the same benefits. The chart demonstrates that you are not.

All the activities on our list have tangible benefits. Even the very low impact ones are great for reducing stress levels. But in terms of FFB, don't consider them money in the bank.

Comparitive Sports Benefit Chart*

Activity	cardio	strength	flexibility	fat burning	score
Golf	3	3	6	3	15
Tennis	6	6	6	6	24
Skiing/ snowboarding	6	6	6	6	24
Surfing	6	6	6	6	24
Squash	9	6	6	9	30
Cycling	9	6	3	9	27
Rowing	9	6	6	9	30
Paddling (kayak or ski)	9	6	6	9	30
Sailing	3	3	3	3	12
Swimming	9	6	6	6	27
Running	9	3	6	9	27
Aerobics	9	6	6	9	30
Weight lifting	6	9	3	3	21
Power walking	6	3	3	3	15
FFB	9	9	6	9	33

*Comparisons are based on an hour spent on each activity at a competent level of expertise. Fat burning is measured as calories burnt per hour by a person of 70kg. Scores in each category are out of 10 with low range averaged at 3, medium at 6 and high at 9. Activities scoring higher than 20 are good all round conditioning exercises.

Golf

This is a great recreation, and if you walk the 18 holes briskly, you'll get some cardio benefit. Unfortunately too many people ride golf carts and the only exercise they get is swinging the club or opening the beer on the way to the next tee.

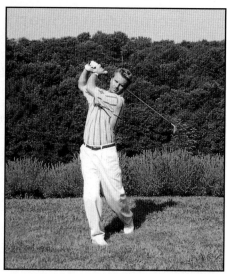

Tennis

Again, the benefits vary according to how you play the game. For the purposes of comparison, we're assuming an hour of singles played at a reasonable level of competence, but as any social tennis player will attest, this still leaves a lot of variance. Some social players will hunt a ball down relentlessly, regardless of their ability to hit it back, while other better players will draw the line at diving or scrambling to the net. The more ball chasing you do, the better the aerobic workout. Tennis also offers a good anaerobic workout with plenty of explosive starts in order to retrieve shots.

While the game doesn't offer much for all-round strength, it is very good for leg development. In fact, if you combined a couple of solid games of tennis with your FFB programs each week, you'd have a very good all-round program.

Skiing/Snowboarding

Great for lower body strength and a good cardiovascular workout as well. If you're snowboarding and using lifts you're not going to get much upper body benefit. Downhill skiers put in some shoulder work with their stocks, but the real all-round workout in the snow comes when you dispense with all the conveniences of a modern ski resort. Cross country skiers are among the fittest athletes in the world.

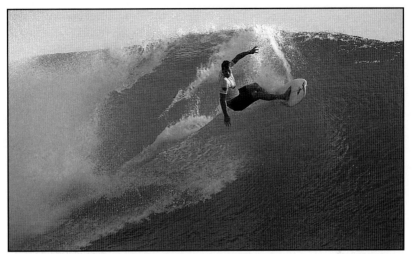

Pro surfer Jeff Booth gets an all-round workout on this powerful Indonesian wave.

Surfing

A very good sport for all-round fitness, with the emphasis on the upper body. Upper body muscle endurance has to be well developed if you are going to paddle after waves for hours at a time, then when you are riding the wave, the lower body gets a pretty good workout too, with a lot of power exerted in turning the board. So you need muscle endurance, power and anaerobic fitness for the legs. Surfing is a quite effective fat burner too.

Squash

Like tennis, the benefits from squash really depend on how hard you play the game. It's high on anaerobic benefit with a lot of sprints over very short distances. The cardiovascular benefit will also be quite high, assuming you play for at least 40 minutes without a long break. Essentially a lower body workout, squash also requires a good deal of all-round flexibility.

Cycling

Recreational cycling is a good fat burner and lower body workout. Mountain biking is a considerably more strenuous (and increasingly popular) form of the sport, providing good cardiovascular benefits as well as lower body. Competitive cycling is a whole different world. Apart from

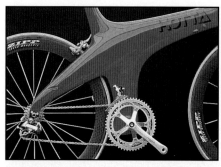

all the drug allegations, the top competitive cyclists I've seen are right up there with cross-country skiers in terms of total fitness.

Rowing

A great all-round workout encompassing co-ordinated movement of both upper and lower body. Rowing can also be a great team sport, with a fantastic social atmosphere amongst motivated people who love to train hard. The downside is that you have to join a club and you are reliant on the availability of others to train. And going it alone in rowing can be a costly exercise.

Paddling (ski or kayak)

Paddling, on the other hand, is tailor-made for the individual. The equipment is relatively inexpensive and can be carried to and from the water by one person. It's great for strength and fat burning, and although the legs aren't utilised as much as in rowing, the cardio and strength gains are great.

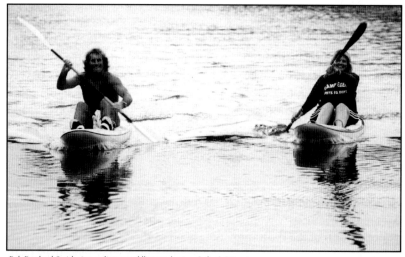

Rob Rowland-Smith gives a client a paddling workout on Sydney's Pittwater.

Sailing

A low impact recreation, unless you're solo sailing a Hobie cat in a gale. A grinder on an America's Cup crew gets a pretty good workout too, but between those two extremes, pleasure sailing is a great way to spend a sunny afternoon and not much of a workout. However, for stress relief sailing is hard to beat.

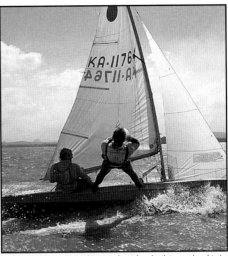

This is a workout: any sailing you do with a drink in one hand isn't.

Swimming

High cardiovascular activity using all muscle groups. The beauty of swimming is that it's so low impact, with very little injury risk. The negative is that you have to spend much longer at it than most other sports to derive the benefits. If you're a lap swimmer using a full range of strokes the benefit to strength and flexibility is very high.

Running

Two different energy systems come into play in running. Sprinting is a good anaerobic activity with limited cardiovascular benefit. Distance running, which is what most recreational runners prefer, is a fat burner and a great cardio workout. If you vary the surface and the scenery, you'll get more of a lower body workout and you'll be less likely to get bored.

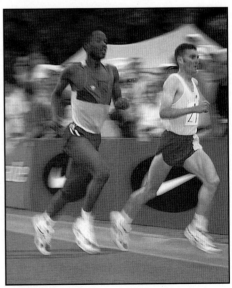

Aerobics

Fantastic cardiovascular workout and, depending on what variation you choose, it can also be a very good all-round workout. "Pump", which employs weights, is probably the best type of aerobics for all-round fitness.

Weightlifting

The benefits depend entirely on why you are lifting weights. If you want to develop power and build muscle mass you will be lifting heavy weights in short repetitions with long recovery periods. This will certainly increase strength but there is very little cardiovascular benefit. Circuit training, with continuous activity using lighter weights, is a very good cardio workout.

Power walking

Power walking and hiking are a gear or two down from running but they are enjoyable and worthwhile, particularly for people who find it difficult to run for sustained periods. Again, time is a major factor. To achieve the same fat burning benefits as an hour of running, you would need to walk for two hours.

FFB

Our program simply puts all the benefits into one time-effective package. We aren't suggesting that FFB is better than all the other activities listed; only that it is designed to maximise all fitness benefits in the space of one hour. The ideal scenario would be to use FFB as your fitness insurance and then try to make time to enjoy four or five of the other medium to high benefit activities.

Chapter 7

Living Proof

Harry

Since I began the Fit For Business program in earnest in December 1997 I've been very pleased with the results. Okay, it hasn't given me the body form of a 20-year-old, or even a 30-year-old, but the body fat loss and lean muscle gain have been reward enough.

Most important, however, is how I feel. The all-round fitness level that FFB has given me is the most pleasing aspect, and one in which I take considerable pride. Just three years back I would stand around at the events my company sponsors (surfing, windsurfing and snowboarding) and feel intimidated by the athletes who were competing. In most cases these guys were 25 years younger than me and gifted with rare natural talent in their chosen sport, so obviously there wasn't going to be any catching up! But I just felt a little disappointed in myself that the course of my life had led me so far away from the level of fitness I had always aspired to.

Often at these events I would also see Rob Rowland-Smith, our international team fitness trainer, and that would depress me even more! Not that Rob is a depressing person to have around - quite the opposite - but here was a contemporary of mine, fitter and stronger than 90% of the young athletes he trained. It was at one of these events that I finally asked Rob to work with me on a specialised training program for people like me.

Since then the rewards of FFB have given me a new confidence in myself and I now feel totally at ease in the company of the sporting champions with whom I deal in business on a daily basis. I can't do what they do, but like Rob, I'm as fit or fitter than they are, and I'm given due respect for that achievement. After the analysis of my results from the fitness testing that Rob, publisher Phil Jarratt and I underwent in Sydney, it became clear to all of us involved in FFB that the program not only achieved our objectives, it far exceeded them. Since then we've been demonstrating FFB to the world - well, our world at least - in the hope that through constructive and objective criticism we could iron out any wrinkles.

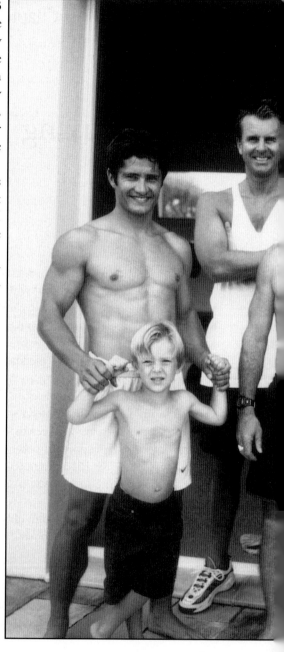

"They'll all be 50 one day too!" Our FFB champion testing panel outside my home gym in Bidart. Left to right: soccer star Bixente Lizarazu (with my son Tommy); surfing champions Tom Carroll and Kelly Slater; windsurfing champion Robby Naish.

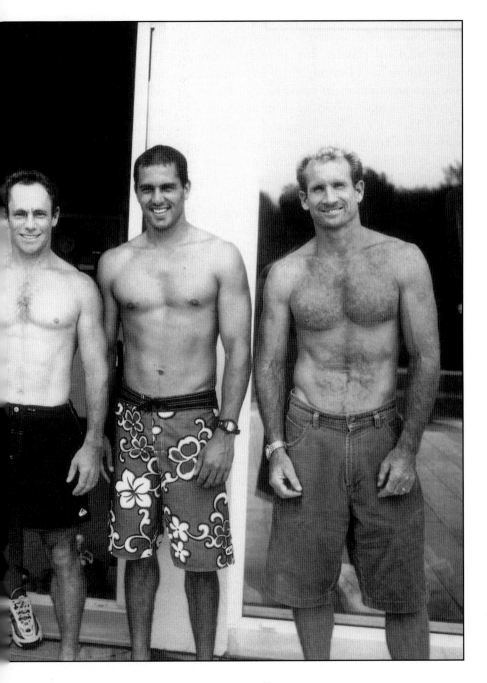

For me this process has been very enjoyable, allowing me to turn a lot of friends on to FFB. Of course our program is designed specifically for busy working people, not sporting champions, but I felt that endorsement from elite athletes (who have access to every conditioning program known to man) would be the icing on the cake for FFB.

Twenty-four-times world windsurfing champion Robby Naish, from Oahu, Hawaii, is a close friend and a sporting phenomenon. Since his early teen years he has dominated his chosen sport, while at the same time developing into an all-round waterman in the classic Hawaiian tradition. There is nothing on water that this guy cannot do! Twice world surfing champion Tom Carroll, from Sydney, Australia, is another phenomenon. Since winning his world titles in the early 1980s, Tom has placed greater emphasis on fitness training (Rob says he is the fittest and most dedicated sportsman he has ever worked with) so that now, in his mid-30s, he is fitter than he was at his competitive peak and surfing better than ever. In 1999 he entered the Masters ranks with form good enough for him to still be competing on the main World Championship Tour.

I have trained with both these guys (together and separately) at my home gym and at workout centres around the world. Since we developed FFB they have both tried the program and now incorporate it into their training schedules.

Robby : "I've done the Fit For Business program a number of times now and it amazes me how efficient and beneficial it is when you consider how little time you spend working out. For a businessman or woman I can't imagine a better workout program. As a professional athlete I know the benefits of training and staying in shape, but what Harry has done with the FFB program shows that physical fitness can cross over into mental fitness. Since he started doing the program he's really taken control, handling the stresses and pressures of business better than ever before."

Tom: "Fit For Business is a great pump-up! I've been doing super-sets for a long time now, but the way they're put together in this program is a really good workout. Since I've put FFB into my overall program I've increased my strength, particularly in my back, my posture is better and I feel better."

I have also introduced six-times world surfing champion Kelly Slater to the program and he has trained with me on several occasions. At 27 he is considered one of the most naturally fit athletes in the world, but he found FFB beneficial and even challenging, stimulating a few muscle groups he'd been neglecting.

My fitness test results for anaerobic capacity underline the fact that FFB is a solid grounding for all kinds of athletic activity, but I was nonetheless very pleased and proud when my friend, French World Cup soccer star Bixente Lizarazu agreed to try out the program. Bixente, in the prime of his career, plays for top European club Bayern Munich as well as for France, and he works tirelessly on his fitness level to ensure he does not lose his competitive edge in an extremely competitive sport.

When I outlined the FFB program to him, he expressed some misgivings about the weights routines, but agreed to try it anyway. He rode his bike 15 kilometres from his place to mine as a warm-up, then did the full program with me. He said: "I think the concept is very good because you can train for your heart and your muscle groups at the same time. You can improve your physical condition without putting stress on your body, which makes it a great program for everyone."

Next evening we were at dinner with French tennis star Guy Forget and I overheard Bixente extolling the virtues of FFB to Guy. That gave me a great sense of pride, to know that sporting champions of such calibre would be interested in a program we had devised for normal businessmen and women.

But the real proof of FFB's value will be in its reception from the people for whom it was devised. So, as we put the finishing touches on this book during the European summer of 1999, I invited some of my business associates to try the program and comment. Some of these people were basically unfit in early middle age, and they found FFB a major challenge. We took it slowly and made sure they adopted correct technique, but in several cases I could see that the will to attain a higher level of fitness was not yet great. A few more years and a few more kilos, I thought, then we'll see. And I hoped that the catalyst for them to start thinking about fitness would not be anything more serious than a spare tyre around the middle!

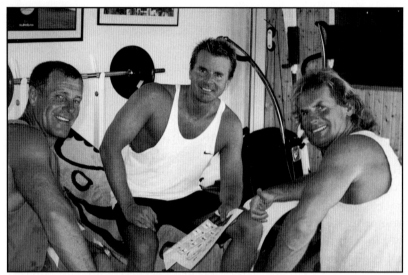

Above: acquainting Toni Vanderwalle with FFB. Below: Toni and Harry at work on a super-set.

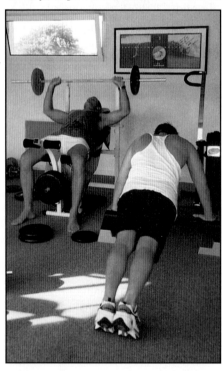

More beneficial for both parties were the trial FFB sessions I initiated with business acquaintances I knew to have attained a good level of fitness already. Belgian businessman Toni Vandewalle was a classic case. At 40, Toni is Belgium's leading clothing distributor. His company, D'light is a major client of ours and I see him on a regular basis, so I knew how serious he was about his sports - surfing, windsurfing, snowboarding, cycling, golf to name a few - and about retaining his fitness level. But I also knew that he suffered from tendonitis and avoided gym workouts. Getting him to try

FFB wasn't difficult, but the moment he entered the gym I knew he was sceptical.

Rob and I put Toni through a solid FFB workout, taking care not to tax his upper body with too-heavy weights. (There is no greater deterrent than muscles you simply can't use for two days after an initial workout. Sure, all beginners are going to experience some slight muscle soreness, but if it is too painful to work out the next day, then you are trying too hard.) Because he had never used weights, Toni's upper body strength was below what you would expect from looking at him, but in most areas his fitness level enabled him to perform the routines well.

Over a well-earned beer at the conclusion of the workout, he said: "I'm very impressed with FFB. Even the weights part of the program makes a lot of sense, and I've always been sceptical of weights. This was quite different from any workout I've done previously, and I can feel that I've worked my entire body. Any program that can make you feel that way has to be considered worthwhile. I think it will be a good alternative to the swimming and running I already do, and I'll certainly be using FFB, particularly during winter."

Rob

The principles that guide Fit For Business were established long before Harry and I started designing specific programs for business people. They are the principles I have used in my training sessions ever since my early days at the Kings School, and which I have adapted for all kinds of clients, ranging from elite athletes to disabled people or people in rehabilitation from serious injury.

But the embryo that finally became FFB is a group session I have been conducting for several years in the beautiful setting of Sydney's Domain Park. Dubbed "Pain In The Domain" by its participants, this weekday lunchtime cross training workout is not FFB, but it is pretty close. We use bodyweight instead of weights, and a park instead of a gym, but the basic idea is the same - to give the people who really need it a total body workout in a limited time frame.

The Pain crew is drawn from the vocations you find in the "big end of town". They are stockbrokers, merchant bankers, accountants and

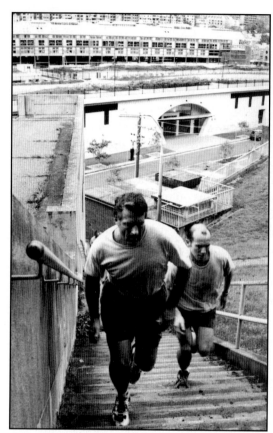

Stair work in the Domain.

lawyers. Some are still active sportsmen, some just have memories and trophy cabinets. But they are all united in their desire to retain their fitness despite the pressures of work. I asked a few of them to explain how they felt about their sessions with the Sandhill Warrior.

Tim Smart

I'm a stock analyst for BT Alex Brown. In winter I play rugby for University of NSW where I've been a member of the Firsts for the past seven years. In summer I play social cricket and golf and I enjoy body surfing, so there are plenty of reasons for me to want to maintain my fitness.

I'm an office worker and generally desk-bound, so it's easy to find that I've finished the day with virtually no exercise. When you combine that lifestyle with regular lunches and business functions, it's easy to fall into a cycle of obesity and lack of fitness. My experience has been that whenever I allow myself to fall into this cycle, my overall alertness, enthusiasm and wellbeing are all affected.

I've tried using a city gym during the week, but I found the atmosphere sterile and the exercises repetitive. Rob Rowland-Smith's sessions in the Domain, on the other hand, are challenging and varied. As a result, I look forward to the sessions, rather than dreading the next trip to the gym. Just as my concentration and enthusiasm for the task at hand begins to wane at the end of the morning, the sessions revitalise both body and mind. Since I joined the group I've noticed a dramatic change in my attentiveness and enthusiasm for work, particularly straight after the sessions. Even in the late afternoons, when I'm accustomed to feeling a little tired and stale, I'm now raring to go.

The variation is one of the most pleasing aspects of Rob's sessions. Just as we've pumped the upper body, we're off doing stair runs, forcing the heart to work harder to push blood back into the legs. This constant variation means that the body is never allowed to settle into a cruising rhythm. It also means that in the course of a session no body part is neglected, and at the end of each workout I feel I've worked on my total fitness.

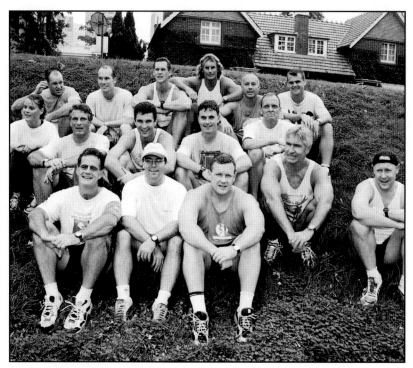

Pain in the Domain crew.

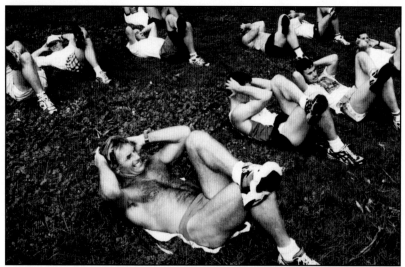

Abs session with the Pain in the Domain crew.

John Campbell

I'm in charge of the Equity Proprietary Trading division at Bankers Trust
Australia. In the past, when work has gotten busy and the family
demanding, the first thing I've tended to abandon has been fitness.
Sometimes I think I was just looking for an excuse! I guess my problem
with training has always been that it just wasn't fun or inspiring, now
that the Olympics are off my agenda.

Since I joined the Sandhill Warrior's band of disciples, my attitude to,
and my enjoyment of fitness has changed. I look forward to it. I find it
fun. I feel better. It breaks up the day and allows me to totally forget
about things for an hour or so.

Training with a group helps me enormously, so much so that even when
things get tough at work I find I can maintain my fitness regime to some
degree. I'm not the fittest in the group but I don't care. All I'm after is
something that's fun and helps me to maintain my body and mind at a
reasonable level in the face of the immutable laws of gravity and entropy.
Is there a better trainer than Rob Rowland-Smith? Possibly. Is there a
better motivator? Unlikely.

Chris Haynes
Vice-President, BT Alex Brown

12.45 Monday and Wednesday, be there
The Sandhill Warrior comes to town with his long locks of hair
Merchant bankers, lawyers, accountants come all
It's that time of the week to get out of your stall
Pasty white skin and coffee cuisine
Test themselves against the man from down past Narrabeen
Bodies who for the rest of the week are at desks
Now restoration begins, hopefully back to their best.
350 situps to start, we begin at gentlemen's pace,
Let's get fit, says the warrior as the grimaces appear on our face.
For the next hour and a half who knows what's in store?
There is one thing for certain, we are going to be sore...

(Don't give up your day job, Chris.-RRS)

Damian Kelly
I head up Salomon Smith Barney Futures and I'm happily married with four children under four! I've been heavily involved in sport from a very early age and as a result always managed to maintain a good level of fitness. Consequently I never ever thought I would need the services of a personal trainer (God forbid!), until that period in my life when I started to think that work was more important than anything else in my life, and if I was exercising, I wasn't working.

I soon became overweight, unfit and unhappy. I started to lose motivation at work, I lost confidence in myself and my self esteem was not what it should be to be successful in life. All the work I'd put in was starting to seem like a waste of time.

When I met Rob I sensed immediately that my life was going to change. I knew that this wasn't a fit guy killing time between vocations, but rather a fitness professional who could see what I needed to pull myself out of the rut. He started helping me do that from the very first session. My wife often jokes that I become a pain in the proverbial if I miss a single session with Rob, and it's true. I've

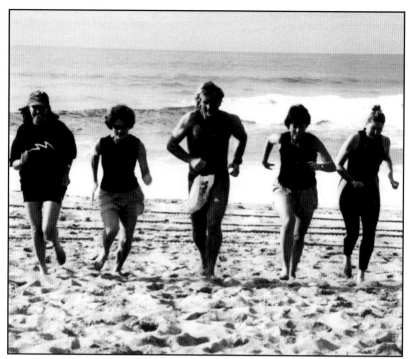

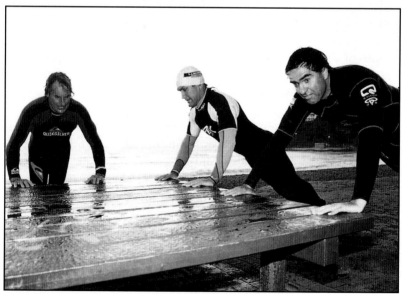

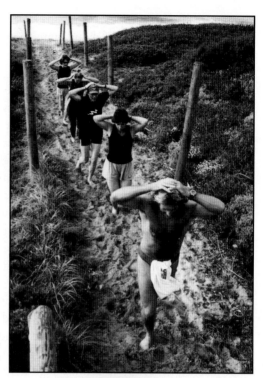

Living proof! Rob puts his crews through their paces. Opposite page and right: The Palm Beach girls' group. Below: Palm Beach mens' group.

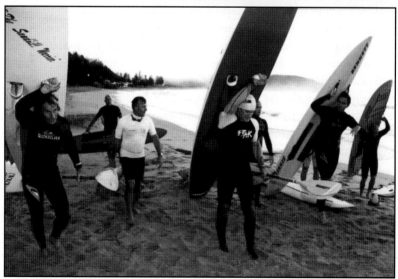

come to realise how important it is to have that balance in your life. I no longer have to worry about motivating myself to train. Rob has done that permanently.

While all these people are for me the real "living proof" of the effectiveness of fitness training within a busy working life, we had to look no further than our editor and publisher Phil Jarratt for proof that FFB will work on even the most hardened cases of sedentary excess.

I'm overstating the case here a bit, for as a lifelong surfer and dedicated jogger (with one marathon and a bunch of fun runs under his belt), Phil had always been active to some degree, doing some form of exercise three to four times a week year-round. However, he was the first to admit that the kind of exercise he did - jogging on the beach one day, an hour in the surf the next - was not working his entire body and was certainly not keeping pace with a busy working life which involves lots of travel and many social functions.

Phil began dabbling in FFB as we worked on this book in France in the summer of 1998, working out with Harry and me for a couple of weeks at a time. But he was not consistent with it and certainly not committed to the program. Therefore when it came time to do our fitness testing in Sydney in April 1999, it seemed logical to have Phil tested as the "before", a role which he accepted with only marginal discomfort. His results (detailed in Chapter 1) revealed a typical case of a businessman in middle age who had the will to be fit but not the methodology. His aerobic capacity was above average (thanks to the running) and he could pull heavy weight (thanks to the surfboard paddling) but not push it. His abdominal strength was well below average since he hated sit-ups and hadn't developed the discipline of a well-organised training program.

As businessmen of similar age, one having done FFB, the other not, Phil and Harry's fitness test results provided an interesting contrast, and pointed to the many areas of fitness that FFB addresses which are overlooked in other programs or sporting activities. But the real proof of the effectiveness of FFB came when Phil looked at the test results and immediately made a commitment to the program. In the six months since then he has averaged more than four FFB workouts a week, and has begun to incorporate soft sand beach sessions, forest runs and mountain

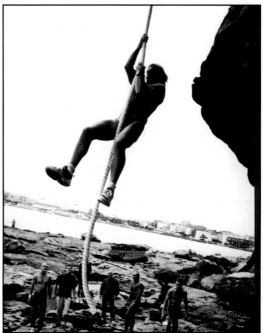

Working with the Bondi crew.

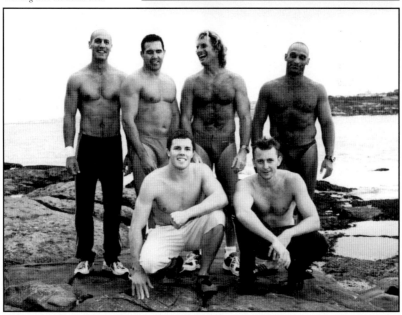

biking as well as his regular surfing. At 48, his body has begun to tone up, he has lost some of the weight around his middle and stacked it on his shoulders. He has a long way to go, but he feels much better, he functions much better at work and at home, and, most importantly, he is firmly committed to FFB.

On one of our weekend editing sessions at Phil's home in Noosa Heads, Queensland, Phil asked me to introduce his friend, local restaurateur and businessman Lyndon Simmons, to the joys of FFB. At the age of 50, Simmo is trim, lean and strong, the result of an everyday exercise regime which includes swimming the length of Noosa's Main Beach. He had gym memberships and used them occasionally but, like many people, he found the machinery confusing and the workouts difficult to manage.

We put Simmo through a good FFB session in the gym at the Sheraton Noosa Resort. His verdict: "Well, at last a workout that makes sense!" Then we made plans to do it all again the next day. Come the morning, Simmo was a no-show. He had all sorts of excuses, but it didn't matter. He's tasted FFB, we'll get him in the end.

Chapter 8

Using Fit For Business

A user friendly guide to your FFB charts

Rob

The seven charts included in this book will guide you through every step of the Fit For Business program. The information on each chart will explain the function of each exercise, but please take the time to read through this guide so that you understand exactly how to proceed with the program for maximum benefit and enjoyment. Here we will also explain which muscle group is being worked and to what benefit.

The first chart is a guide to warming up your body in preparation for the program. You should complete both the stretches and the light weights routine before proceeding with each FFB program. Also use the stretches to "stretch down" after completing each workout.

The last chart details the abdominal exercise routine you should follow after completing the 10 FFB exercises, plus some ancillory exercises that may be done when the equipment is available. These ancillory exercises are also a great way to add variety to your program, as well as providing an extra challenge.

The five FFB programs use a total of 29 different exercises in 100 sets (or 50 supersets). They are designed to work every muscle group during each workout, and to provide variety of routine so that you are not faced with exactly the same workout each day. This variety stimulates fitness development and muscle growth as the challenge of the program changes on a daily basis. The programs numbered one to five are not graded progressively, however beginners should start using very light weights and aim to work upward. The standard workout for males is three sets of 12/10/8 repetitions, for females 15/12/10 using lighter weights. However beginners should progress slowly, doing one set of 12 or 15 repetitions for the first cycle of programs, then doing two sets of 12/10 or 15/12 repetitions for the second cycle. If limited weights are available (ie. too heavy or too light) adjust repetitions accordingly. Always remember to work within your limits when using weights. If you can't do the repetitions then the weight is too heavy. Don't push yourself too hard, and always remember that when using weights correct technique is essential. Bend your knees and pick up weights with a straight back. Picking up weights with straight legs and rounded back can lead to serious injury. Make sure that the weight plates are secured by collars. Ensure that the weight plates are evenly distributed.

The FFB program has been designed for maximum time-efficiency. Under normal conditions, you should be able to complete the entire workout (including stretches at either end) within one hour. Two people can effectively share the same equipment within this time frame, however it's possible for three to use one set of equipment with the third partner running on the spot between exercises and "spotting" to ensure safety when using weights. Quite often the group session is a fun way of training and can inspire greater motivation to perform.

One of the great advantages of FFB is that you can do the program just about anywhere at any time. If finding time is your major problem, this can mean eliminating cross-town hikes to the gym. Your garage or den at home can be a totally adequate substitute for a fully-equipped gymnasium with just a little bit of improvisation. Even your hotel room can provide enough space to work out, with chairs or TV benches pressed into service as training equipment. By combining the bodyweight exercises in your FFB programs, you can even have a profitable workout without the use of weights. Just use your imagination.

Stretches

A warm-up 1) increases body temperature, 2) increases respiration and heart rate, and 3) guards against muscle, tendon and ligament strains. It is also an opportunity to prepare mentally for the workout ahead.

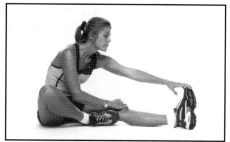

During this light activity, set your goals and plan your approach to each exercise. For example, if you've been having difficulty with the bench press, focus on your technique during warm-up, so that is fresh in your mind when you apply it. The cool-down is just as important as the warm-up. An abrupt finish to your workout can lead to pooling of the blood, sluggish circulation and the slow removal of waste products. The cool-down helps lower the body temperature and bring down the heart rate.

To gain maximum value from stretching, it is important to follow the sequence of exercises, and to hold each exercise for at least 15 seconds.

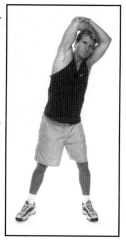

Light Weights Warm-Up

The light weights routine is essentially a dress rehearsal for the FFB program. The idea is to stimulate blood flow to the muscles and to raise the heart rate a little further. Use light weights - ideally dumbells between 2.5 and 5kg. If you have to use a barbell, it should be between 7.5kg and 10kg. The use of too-heavy weights in this part of the program will inhibit your ability to work at full capacity during the rest of FFB.

Perform this routine continuously, moving from one exercise to the next in an easy flow of movement. Give yourself 30 seconds to recover between each set.

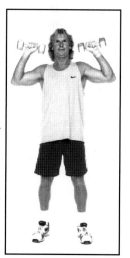

FFB Program 1

Superset 1.

Barbell bench press super-setted with normal push-up.

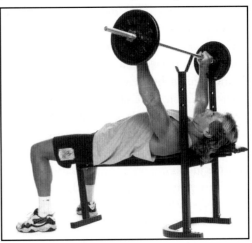

The bench press is the core exercise for the upper body. It stimulates all upper body muscles. Lie on your back on the bench, feet flat, arms slightly wider than shoulder width. Take the bar off the rack and extend upwards. It is important to breathe out when pushing the weight up. Do this exercise in a controlled manner, and when replacing the weight ensure that your hands are clear of the support rack. When lifting heavier weights, use a partner to "spot" for you.

Like the bench press, the push-up is the core bodyweight exercise for strength and development of the upper body. The placement of hands for the normal push-up is just outside the shoulders. It is important to keep the back straight and lower down until the chest touches the floor.

Superset 2.

Dumbell incline bench press super-setted with decline push-up.

Do this press on an incline bench at a 45 degree angle. The dumbells are facing each other at shoulder height. Push them upwards and turn them out. This exercise stimulates the upper chest, shoulder and tricep area.

The decline push-up stimulates the lower half of the chest, as well as tricep and upper shoulder. Keep your feet 6-8" apart on step or bench and lower the body until the chest touches the floor. The higher the step or bench, the greater the efficiency of the exercise. Think about your breathing and exhale on the downward movement.

Superset 3.
Barbell curl super-setted with close-hand incline push-up.

The barbell curl works the upper arm and bicep area. Stand erect, feet comfortably apart and knees slightly flexed. Hold the bar in front of the thighs with an underhand grip, with the hands shoulder-width apart. Flex the elbows, lifting bar towards chest. Do not lean backwards or bounce the bar. Beginners should lean against a wall to learn the correct technique and prevent injury.

The close-hand incline push-up works the tricep muscles and the inner range of the chest. The tricep forms the major part of the upper arm. Exhale on the downward movement.

Superset 4.
Dumbell tricep extension super-setted with tricep dip.

The dumbell tricep extension really isolates the tricep muscle. Sit at the end of the bench, feet shoulder width apart and back straight. Take the dumbell behind the head with your hands forming a triangle around the base of the plate. Keeping your elbows as close to the head as possible, extend the dumbell. Take care when initially placing the dumbell behind your head and do not swing to the side. Do this exercise in a controlled manner.

Tricep dips work the upper back as well as the triceps. Hands should be shoulder-width apart, facing outward. Lower the body without touching the floor, then extend arms.

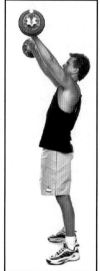

Superset 5.
Barbell military press (standing) super-setted with incline push-up.

The military press is a great shoulder development exercise as it stimulates all parts of the deltoid area. Grasp the barbell with an overhand grip, then press the barbell overhead at 45 degrees until the elbows are fully extended. Lower the bar to chest position.

The incline push-up works the upper chest and deltoid area. Position as per 3 but with hands at shoulder width.

Superset 6.
Barbell upright row super-setted with wide-arm push-up.
The upright rowing exercise must be done with the hands close together to stimulate the shoulders and upper back. The key to this exercise is to draw the bar to the chin with the elbows higher than the shoulders. Keep your back straight and feet shoulder-width apart.

The wide-arm push-up without the incline stimulates the shoulders and upper back.

Superset 7.
Dumbell single-arm row super-setted with one-arm incline push-up.
Whereas the upright rowing movement stimulates the upper back around the shoulder region, this movement stimulates the lats, which are the big muscles on the side of the back. Place one knee on the bench, extend one arm to support the upper body and draw the weight upwards with a very high elbow. It is imperative to keep the back straight.

The one-arm incline push-up also stimulates this muscle group. It is important to get the feet placement correct to allow for a full range of movement. Feet placement in both these exercises is similar.

Superset 8.
Leg extension super-setted with butt bounce.
The leg extension works primarily the quadricep area. (These are the four muscles that form the upper thigh.) Sit at the end of the bench, placing lower legs under the crossbar. Extend upwards. (When purchasing your multi-purpose bench, be sure that it includes a leg extension/leg curl facility.)

The butt bounce works the quadricep/hamstring (muscles behind the back of the leg)/ butt. Adopt a push-up position, extend one leg backwards. Do a bounce movement. Repeat with other leg. When counting the repetitions make sure that the full sequence is done for each leg.

Superset 9.
Leg curl super-setted with lateral extension.
The leg curl works the hamstring muscles at the back of the upper thigh. Lie face down on the bench with heels positioned behind the padded

bar. Flex the legs to elevate the weight and then return to starting position. Lateral extensions work the inner muscles of the upper thigh. Adopt a wide stance and drop body weight with elbow resting on knee. The other arm should support the upper body. Move sideways, reversing the position. Make sure you do the full sequence for each side.

Superset 10.
Dumbell half-squat super-setted with butt raise.
Like the bench press, the squat is the core exercise for the lower body. It works all the muscles of the legs, the lower back area and the butt. Hold the dumbells by your side, keeping your back straight and your feet wide, lower your body to a position just below parallel. Be sure to keep your arms straight at all times. Push upwards and breathe out. Do not have a rounded back as this could lead to injury.

The butt raise movement is a direct opposite to the squat. Your feet are shoulder-width apart, you are leaning forward, your elbows keep the knees parallel with your fingers interlocked, ie, a crouch position. Raise the butt without moving the lower leg or the arms.

FFB Program 2

Superset 1.
Dumbell flat bench press super-setted with normal push-up.
This dumbell press is similar to the bench press. The advantage of using dumbells is that you work a wider range of movement. Lie flat on the bench, push the dumbells upwards and turn inwards midway.
Push-up as per Program 1.

Superset 2.
Barbell incline bench press super-setted with decline push-up.
The incline barbell bench press is similar to the dumbell press used in

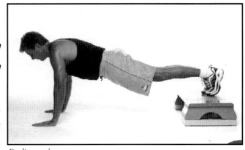

Decline push-up.

Program 1. The muscle groups exercised are exactly the same as for dumbells. With the barbell, however, you use a wider grip, therefore stimulating the outside muscles of the chest. When increasing the weight, make sure that you have a "spotter" to help you.
Decline push-up as per Program 1.

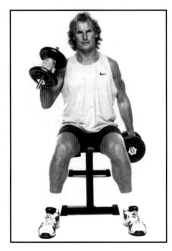

Superset 3.
Dumbell hammer curl super-setted with incline push-up.
Use dumbells for the hammer curl. This exercise not only works the upper arm but the fore-arms too. Sit at the end of the bench with feet slightly wider than shoulder-width, hold dumbells by your sides and alternately lift through full range of movement.
Incline push-up as per Program 1 but hands at shoulder-width.

Superset 4.
Dumbell tricep extension super-setted with tricep dip.
As per Program 1.

Superset 5.
Seated dumbell punch super-setted with wide hand push-up.
Sit at the end of the bench with your back straight and feet shoulder-width apart. Lift the dumbells to shoulder height and push alternately in the air.
Wide hand floor push-ups as per Program 1.

Superset 6.
Barbell upright row super-setted with wide-hand incline push-up.
As per Program 1.

Superset 7.
Dumbell single-arm row super-setted with one-arm incline push-up.
As per Program 1.

Superset 8.
Leg extension super-setted with butt bounce.
As per Program 1.

Superset 9.
Dumbell lunge super-setted with butt raise.
The dumbell lunge is a great exercise for the butt and upper thigh. Pick up the dumbells as you would for the dumbell half-squat, keeping your feet shoulder-width apart. Keeping your back straight lunge forward, dropping to parallel. Do this exercise with each leg working alternately, with full range of movement on each leg.
Butt raises as per Program 1.

Superset 10.
Dumbell calf raise super-setted with lateral extension.
With straight arms hold the dumbells alongside your upper thighs in an upright standing position. Curl up onto your toes, pause for a second, then repeat the movement. For a more advanced movement place a weight plate underneath each set of toes and do the calf-raise movement using the weight to give you a greater range of movement. Lateral extensions as per Program 1.

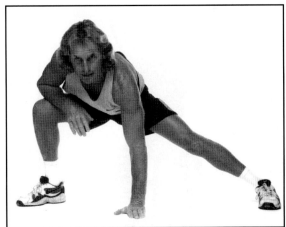

Program 3

All exercises as described in previous programs unless otherwise stated.

Superset 1.
Barbell flat bench press super-setted with normal push-up.

Superset 2.
Flat bench dumbell press super-setted with decline push-up.

Superset 3.
Barbell curl super-setted with close-hand incline push-up.

Superset 4.
Dumbell tricep extension super-setted with tricep dip.

Superset 5.
Barbell seated press behind neck super-setted with wide-arm push-up.

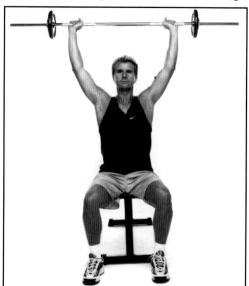

The press behind neck stimulates the back of the shoulder, back of neck and upper back. Position yourself at the end of bench with feet slightly wider than shoulder-width, position weight behind the head and extend upwards. Initially this exercise may require a "spotter".

Superset 6.

Barbell upright row super-setted with wide-arm incline push-up.

Superset 7.

Dumbell single-arm row super-setted with one-arm incline push-up.

Superset 8.

Dumbell half-squat super-setted with butt raise.

Superset 9.

Leg curl super-setted with lateral extension.

Superset 10.

Dumbell lunge super-setted with butt bounce.

Program 4

Superset 1.

Barbell close-grip bench press super-setted with close-hand incline push-up.

This press works the tricep and inner range of chest area. Lie flat on the bench and take a close grip of the bar inside the uprights. Lower bar to chest and push upwards.

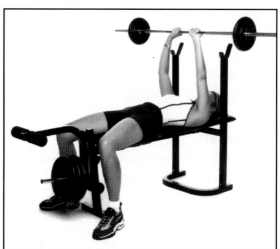

Superset 2.
Dumbell incline bench press super-setted with decline push-up.

Superset 3.
Dumbell hammer curl super-setted with incline push-up.

Superset 4.
Dumbell tricep extension super-setted with tricep dip.

Superset 5.
Barbell upright row super-setted with wide-arm incline push-up.

Superset 6.
Barbell military press (standing) super-setted with wide-arm push-up.

Superset 7.
Dumbell single-arm row super-setted with one-arm incline push-up.

Superset 8.
Leg extension super-setted with butt raise.

Superset 9.
Dumbell lunge super-setted with lateral extension.

Superset 10.
*Dumbell bench step super-setted with half-squat
(hands on hips, no weight).*
Hold dumbells at sides and step onto bench, alternating lead foot.
To do the half-squat place your feet wider than shoulder-width, place
hands on hips and squat to parallel.

Program 5

Superset 1.
Barbell bench press super-setted with normal push-up.

Superset 2.
Barbell Incline bench press super-setted with decline push-up.

Superset 3.
Barbell curl super-setted with close-hand incline push-up.

Superset 4.
Dumbell tricep extension super-setted with tricep dip.

Superset 5.
Barbell upright row super-setted with wide-arm incline push-up.

Superset 6.
Barbell seated press behind neck super-setted with wide-arm push-up.

Superset 7.
Dumbell single-arm row super-setted with single-arm push-up.

Superset 8.
Leg curl super-setted with butt bounce.

Superset 9.
Dumbell bench step super-setted with butt raise.

Superset 10.
Calf raise super-setted with lateral extension.

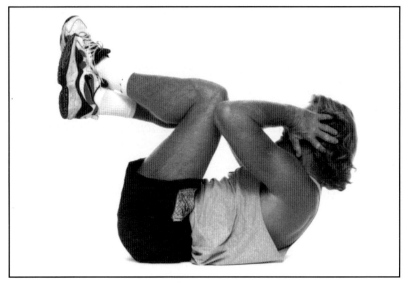

Abdominals

I've always believed that the abdominals are the most important muscle group in the body. The abdominal area is where we twist, turn and pivot from in a whole range of day-to-day activities. As we get older and gravity takes over it is very easy to lose the tone and strength in the mid-range of the body. This can lead to lower back problems which can be avoided or rectified through strengthening of the abdominals. More than 30 million Americans are afflicted with lower back pain and an estimated 80% of these problems are due to bad posture and weak muscle development in the abdominals. The abdominals are a muscle group that can be exercised daily, anywhere, any time.

It is important when working the abdominals to adhere strictly to the instructions on the chart. Beginners should start by doing 10 repetitions of each of the five exercises. If you feel you can do more, repeat the set. FFB users should be aiming to work up to a full set of 500 as soon as possible. Do these exercises in a slow and controlled manner, concentrating at all times on contracting the abdominal muscles as you go through the movement. Breathing is just as important as body position. Don't cut corners in this workout because it comes at the end of the program. And remember, while it is relatively easy to fake an abs workout, you are only fooling yourself.

Ancillory Exercises.

No matter how fit and strong we think we are, there is always a greater challenge. I have always believed that power-to-bodyweight ratio is the greatest indicator of strength and muscle endurance. As you proceed through the FFB programs you are not only going to get fitter and leaner, but also ultimately stronger. Try then to incorporate the bodyweight ancillary exercises described in the chart. The ability to lift your own bodyweight (ie doing the three different forms of chin-ups and dips) should be seen as the next challenge once you have reached a level of competence in FFB.

The knee raise and hanging leg raise exercises are a great supplement to your abdominal workout. Doing these exercises works not only the abdominals but the hip flexors as well.

For a relatively modest outlay (for a Tower of Power or even a chin bar, plus focus pads and punching mits) you can be equipped to take your training into a new realm.

In conclusion

If some one tells you there's a no-sweat, no-pain way to get fit, it's a lie. If you really want to get results then you have to be consistent and work hard, and at the same time enjoy what you're doing. There's no reward for conning your body. It knows how much effort it's making and it will respond accordingly when it comes to getting fitter and burning fat.

When doing the FFB program, make sure you do the exercises correctly, even if it means cutting back on the weights you are using. Strength and fitness will improve much faster if you do the exercises properly with lighter weights than it will if you let your ego take over and try to lift too much, or if you cheat on the bodyweight exercises by doing half-movements or by doing them too quickly.

If possible, try to train with a partner. By working with some one else who is also keen and has a similar attitude to health and fitness, you will be rewarded with encouragement and inspiration to greater performance. I've always found that consistency is the key element in training, and that quality is much better than quantity when it comes to results. That is the cornerstone of FFB. If you can make FFB a permanent fixture in your lifestyle, we guarantee it will improve your quality of life.

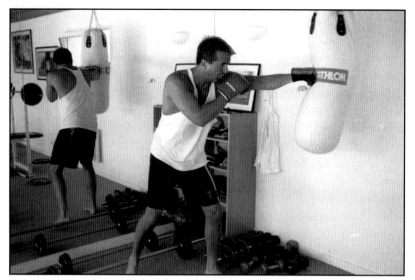

A punching bag warm-up is a good way to vary your FFB workout.

Harry

Working through injuries

One thing I've learnt is that doing any kind of physical exercise you are going to have some minor injuries. Doing a basic fitness program like FFB, you are not likely to suffer any major injury, unless of course you are negligent in using the weights, don't warm up properly or commence the program without a thorough medical check-up first. However, there is a strong likelihood that at some point you will develop some niggling strain. Don't let it sideline you.

Since December 1997 when I embarked upon my FFB journey, I have suffered a back strain and a neck strain from exercise, plus a shoulder injury from snowboarding. And recently I chipped a bone and strained ligaments in my left wrist when I fell over while watering the lawn! All of these were relatively minor injuries, but if I'd been looking for an excuse, they could have sidelined me. Instead, I adopted all the normal techniques of rehabilitation - ice, strap, rest and elevate - and simply worked around them.

We have emphasised throughout this book that correct technique is essential when doing FFB, as it is with any exercise program. I'm therefore a bit embarrassed to admit that my back strain was the result of poor technique and lack of concentration. Because the back is such an important body part I usually go straight to the chiropractor for an expert diagnosis, rather than risk debilitating long-term injury. Once the exact problem has been diagnosed, I then work out how to exercise around the injury, using a weight belt for support and concentrating on bench press exercises where the back is supported.

When I chipped a bone and strained the ligaments in my left wrist, the doctor advised strapping the wrist and having a six-week rest from exercise. Of course I found that unworkable, so I phoned Rob in Australia. Contrary to what the doctor had said, Rob outlined a program that would enable me to keep my fitness level up without exacerbating the injury. I could do pull-ups and chin-ups on the Tower of Power, and I could even do push-ups using a clenched fist. I couldn't lift or push weight but I could still put in a good, if modified, one hour FFB session. My wrist was back to normal in five weeks and I went back to my normal routines. If I'd listened to the doctor I would have been months behind. Elsewhere in this book Rob talks about pro surfer Jeff Booth "parking pain in another room". That's fine when your athletic career is on the line, but people like you and me have jobs to go to and lives to lead. I'm not for a moment suggesting you adopt a gung ho approach when you work out, ignoring the signals your body gives you.

What I am saying is don't use a minor injury as your way out.

Beyond FFB

After 18 months on FFB I've reached the stage where I am looking for ways to "value-add" to FFB. Of course I will never leave the basic programs because I enjoy them so much and know how much they've done to improve my fitness and quality of life. But I always enjoy a new challenge, and for me that now involves constantly adding new activities to my program. I would encourage anyone who has achieved his initial objectives with FFB over a year or more, to keep it interesting through diversification. I do this by sometimes using lighter weights than normal and doing higher repetitions at a faster pace. Basically it's a "Speed FFB" program which takes me about 45 minutes from stretch to stretch, as opposed to

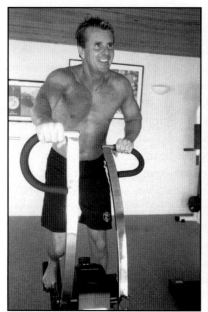 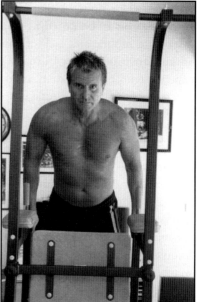

Varying the diet with Cyclone cross trainer and the Tower of Power.

the normal hour. I do this when I'm strapped for time too. The hotel room workout (see box opposite) is another variation that I've added for expediency sake. I try not to stay at hotels that don't have gyms, but it does happen. And when I use hotel gyms, I've also learnt to adapt my program to whatever equipment they have.

At home I've added a Cyclone cross trainer to the "toys" in my gym, plus a Tower of Power and a punching bag. I also have a pool at home and my wife and I do regular aquarobics sessions in the summer months, incorporating running, wading, kicking and swimming. At the beach I've got a whole routine incorporating running on hard sand and soft, shuttle running and wading.

This gives me plenty of variety in my approach to fitness, without resorting to what I regard as high impact activities that can jar ageing bones. I particularly avoid road running, mountain biking and aerobics on hard surfaces.

I have to admit that my favourite place to exercise is my home gym, where I've created a user-friendly environment which works equally well

The Hotel Room Workout

Requirements: enough space to lie down on the floor and extend your arms at right angles; a chair or firm edge at the end of your bed; a raised doorway or some other step.

Stretching: same as for FFB programs, five upper body, five lower, hold each for 10-15 seconds.

1. Push-up and crossed leg push-up (1 set each way). 8/8/8 x 3 sets. Tricep dip and crossed leg tricep dip. 24/24/24 x 3 sets.

2. Decline push-up and crossed leg. 8/8/8 x 3 sets
   Incline push-up and crossed leg. 8/8/8 x 3 sets

3. Wide-arm push-up. 3 sets of 8.
   Incline one-arm push-up. 3 sets of 8.

4. Close hand push-up. 3 sets of 8.
   Close hand tricep dip. 3 sets of 8.

5. Butt raise. 3 sets of 8
   Butt bounce. 3 sets of 8.

6. Bench step (no weights). 3 sets of 8.
   Lateral extension. 3 sets of 8.

7. 90 degree wall squat. 3 sets of 15 seconds.
   Butt bounce. 3 sets of 8.

Abdominals: 500 as per normal FFB.

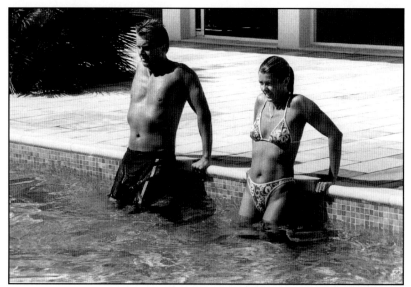

Poolside tricep dips, a summer variation.

for our whole family group or just me. Some people don't like to exercise alone. I love it! After a hard day at the office I'll switch on the TV and catch up with the day's events, or put on some loud '70s rock - The Stones are a favourite - and sweat out my troubles.

You don't need millions to set up a gym like mine, but equally, you can convert any space you have - garage, den, attic or even your backyard - into an FFB world. Make the space work for you and you'll always look forward to your workouts.

Appendix

Monitor Your Progress

The best way to monitor your progress in Fit For Business is to keep a record of your workouts. The mini-diary over the next four pages will allow you to chart your progress during your first year of FFB. Put aside just a few seconds each day to record your workout and calculate your weekly average at the end of each month. Remember that you should aim for five workouts a week and be satisfied with an average of three over a whole year in which there may be work, travel or other interruptions to your program. If you're averaging less than three a week after the first month, make more time for yourself.

We also suggest that you monitor the physical benefits of the program by recording your weight, body fat ratio, chest and waist measurements before you start the program, then at quarterly intervals. But don't expect huge gains after the first quarter. Depending on your fitness level at the starting point (if you've got a lot of fat to burn you'll see immediate results in weight loss), you will probably not see a change in body shape until the end of the second quarter.

	Weight	Body fat	Chest	Waist
Starting point				
After 3 months				
After 6 months				
After 9 months				
After 12 months				

FFB

Month 1	Month 2	Month 3
Day 1	Day 1	Day 1
Day 2	Day 2	Day 2
Day 3	Day 3	Day 3
Day 4	Day 4	Day 4
Day 5	Day 5	Day 5
Day 6	Day 6	Day 6
Day 7	Day 7	Day 7
Day 8	Day 8	Day 8
Day 9	Day 9	Day 9
Day 10	Day 10	Day 10
Day 11	Day 11	Day 11
Day 12	Day 12	Day 12
Day 13	Day 13	Day 13
Day 14	Day 14	Day 14
Day 15	Day 15	Day 15
Day 16	Day 16	Day 16
Day 17	Day 17	Day 17
Day 18	Day 18	Day 18
Day 19	Day 19	Day 19
Day 20	Day 20	Day 20
Day 21	Day 21	Day 21
Day 22	Day 22	Day 22
Day 23	Day 23	Day 23
Day 24	Day 24	Day 24
Day 25	Day 25	Day 25
Day 26	Day 26	Day 26
Day 27	Day 27	Day 27
Day 28	Day 28	Day 28
Day 29	Day 29	Day 29
Day 30	Day 30	Day 30
Day 31	Day 31	Day 31
Comments:	Comments:	Comments:
Weekly Average:	Weekly Average:	Weekly Average:

Month 4

Day 1

Day 2

Day 3

Day 4

Day 5

Day 6

Day 7

Day 8

Day 9

Day 10

Day 11

Day 12

Day 13

Day 14

Day 15

Day 16

Day 17

Day 18

Day 19

Day 20

Day 21

Day 22

Day 23

Day 24

Day 25

Day 26

Day 27

Day 28

Day 29

Day 30

Day 31

Comments:

Weekly Average:

Month 5

Day 1

Day 2

Day 3

Day 4

Day 5

Day 6

Day 7

Day 8

Day 9

Day 10

Day 11

Day 12

Day 13

Day 14

Day 15

Day 16

Day 17

Day 18

Day 19

Day 20

Day 21

Day 22

Day 23

Day 24

Day 25

Day 26

Day 27

Day 28

Day 29

Day 30

Day 31

Comments:

Weekly Average:

Month 6

Day 1

Day 2

Day 3

Day 4

Day 5

Day 6

Day 7

Day 8

Day 9

Day 10

Day 11

Day 12

Day 13

Day 14

Day 15

Day 16

Day 17

Day 18

Day 19

Day 20

Day 21

Day 22

Day 23

Day 24

Day 25

Day 26

Day 27

Day 28

Day 29

Day 30

Day 31

Comments:

Weekly Average:

Month 7	Month 8	Month 9
Day 1	Day 1	Day 1
Day 2	Day 2	Day 2
Day 3	Day 3	Day 3
Day 4	Day 4	Day 4
Day 5	Day 5	Day 5
Day 6	Day 6	Day 6
Day 7	Day 7	Day 7
Day 8	Day 8	Day 8
Day 9	Day 9	Day 9
Day 10	Day 10	Day 10
Day 11	Day 11	Day 11
Day 12	Day 12	Day 12
Day 13	Day 13	Day 13
Day 14	Day 14	Day 14
Day 15	Day 15	Day 15
Day 16	Day 16	Day 16
Day 17	Day 17	Day 17
Day 18	Day 18	Day 18
Day 19	Day 19	Day 19
Day 20	Day 20	Day 20
Day 21	Day 21	Day 21
Day 22	Day 22	Day 22
Day 23	Day 23	Day 23
Day 24	Day 24	Day 24
Day 25	Day 25	Day 25
Day 26	Day 26	Day 26
Day 27	Day 27	Day 27
Day 28	Day 28	Day 28
Day 29	Day 29	Day 29
Day 30	Day 30	Day 30
Day 31	Day 31	Day 31
Comments:	Comments:	Comments:
Weekly Average:	Weekly Average:	Weekly Average:

Month 10

Day 1	
Day 2	
Day 3	
Day 4	
Day 5	
Day 6	
Day 7	
Day 8	
Day 9	
Day 10	
Day 11	
Day 12	
Day 13	
Day 14	
Day 15	
Day 16	
Day 17	
Day 18	
Day 19	
Day 20	
Day 21	
Day 22	
Day 23	
Day 24	
Day 25	
Day 26	
Day 27	
Day 28	
Day 29	
Day 30	
Day 31	

Comments:

Weekly Average:

Month 11

Day 1	
Day 2	
Day 3	
Day 4	
Day 5	
Day 6	
Day 7	
Day 8	
Day 9	
Day 10	
Day 11	
Day 12	
Day 13	
Day 14	
Day 15	
Day 16	
Day 17	
Day 18	
Day 19	
Day 20	
Day 21	
Day 22	
Day 23	
Day 24	
Day 25	
Day 26	
Day 27	
Day 28	
Day 29	
Day 30	
Day 31	

Comments:

Weekly Average:

Month 12

Day 1	
Day 2	
Day 3	
Day 4	
Day 5	
Day 6	
Day 7	
Day 8	
Day 9	
Day 10	
Day 11	
Day 12	
Day 13	
Day 14	
Day 15	
Day 16	
Day 17	
Day 18	
Day 19	
Day 20	
Day 21	
Day 22	
Day 23	
Day 24	
Day 25	
Day 26	
Day 27	
Day 28	
Day 29	
Day 30	
Day 31	

Comments:

Weekly Average:

FFB